HANDS-ON
HEALING

HANDS-ON HEALING

Lewis Harrison

Kensington Books
http://www.kensingtonbooks.com

NOTE: The information offered in this book is for educational purposes. The information offered within is not intended for use in the diagnosis, cure, mitigation, treatment or prevention of any disease. Certain persons considered experts may disagree with one or more of the statements, studies, research reports, opinions and conclusions reported or printed herein. The information enclosed may be of current interest and is offered for educational purposes only.

KENSINGTON BOOKS are published by

Kensington Publishing Corp.
850 Third Avenue
New York, NY 10022

Kensington and the K logo Reg. U.S. Pat. & TM Off.

ISBN 1-57566-361-9

First Kensington Trade Paperback Printing: December, 1998
10 9 8 7 6 5 4 3 2 1

Printed in the United States of America

DEDICATION

To my parents Dorothy and Harold Harrison for bringing me to the path. To my first teacher, Vincent Collura for leading me to the secret door of the path. To Maharaj Charan Singh Ji for opening that door and to Baba Gurinder Singh Ji for reminding me that the door is always visible to those who are looking in the right direction.

ACKNOWLEDGMENTS

Thanks to Adam Whyte, Carolyn Schieren, Wayne Olli-vierre, Regine Constant, Miranda B. Norris and Cory Rodin for assisting in the organizing and editing of the manuscript. To Beverly (Beebo) March for creating an incredible support network and for transcribing the "channeled" information on transformation. To Don Dodd for building a working environment so that this gathering of energies could take place. To Nicki Orange and Frank Coticcelli who were always there to help out on a moment's notice. Thanks to Paul Goldner for his abundance, Nancy Rosanoff for her generosity in shar-ing her knowledge on Intuition, Dr. Daniel J. Wiener for his wisdom and clarity, and to Gloria Maddox for being a shining example of how to live fully no matter what the circumstances. I received tremendous support on various aspects of this "Shaman's vision" through Bill Apfil, Jeff and Jean Wolff, Mark Becker, Dr. Jean Miller, Marlene Goldstein, Brenda Shoshana Lukeman, Linda Collura (who offered invaluable friendship and support to my teacher, Vincent, in the last years of his life), my fiancée Lilia Baris and all my friends at The American Polarity Therapy Association and The National Speakers Association.

My special thanks to Luke Felisbret for his fine illus-trations, Anov Adir and Danielle Lynn Pashko for model-ing for the photographs and to Steve Weinberg for taking them. They all worked under extreme conditions and never lost their smiles. Thanks to my editor at Ken-sington Books, Ann LaFarge, who kept me on schedule and who filled in my limitations with her strengths; and to Noah Lukeman, who never lost faith in the vision behind the project.

SPECIAL NOTE

The drawings numbered 1–5, 32, 51–53, 65 are original drawings by Luke Felisbret based on illustrations by Harlan Tarbell, D.N., and concepts presented in the books *Polarity Therapy*, Vol. I and Vol. II, by Dr. Randolph Stone.

The remaining drawings and photographs are all original in concept. These photographs were taken by Steve Weinberg and the illustrations were done by Luke Felisbret. Some of these are based on aspects of my work that were presented in two of my earlier books, both which are out of print: *Massageworks: A Practical Encyclopedia of Massage Techniques,* co-authored with D. Baloti Lawrence, and *Helping Yourself With Natural Healing.*

CONTENTS

INTRODUCTION

Welcome to Hands-On Healing: Massage the Shaman's Way. This book will open a wonderful world of healing and increased intuition through touch.

Though there is no official definition of Shamanism, this form of self-knowledge and healing is achieved by entering into a unique state of consciousness and then accessing certain information while in this state. At its basic level, Shaman Massage is designed not only to reduce tension and stress, but also to enable you to access your intuition at its most subtle and profound levels and utilize this intuitive sensibility into healing touch. This powerful combination is an integral part of the personal growth and healing process.

When combined, Shamanism and massage are powerful tools for self-knowledge and personal growth. If you are in perfect health and have a healthy life-style, you can use Shaman Massage to maintain your health and wellness. As a longevity tool, Shaman Massage can help to guarantee that you will be as healthy in the future as you are now.

When you apply the Shaman Massage Techniques, you will experience a link-up with an internalized radiant energy. The more these exercises and techniques cause you to identify with the radiant energy, the more you will experience the flow of this energy through your body. There will actually be a sensation of the filling of the mind with light, a sense that the heart has filled with love, and the hands with wisdom and power. You will sense that your life has become richer, simpler, and better than it has ever seemed.

Hands-On Healing is a tool for communing consciously with

your deeper being and allowing it to guide everyday actions while serving others through the power of healing touch. It is a touch tool of perception; that is, it gives you access to the extraordinary powers of perception of your deeper self through the practice and application of fourteen powerful bodywork techniques.

Back in the 1960s people got their massages at health clubs and the only kind of massage or bodywork available involved lots of mineral oil, tapping, cupping and Swedish kneading. Things have changed since then. The wellness, New Age and holistic health movements have grown to a billion-dollar service industry. Even insurance companies have begun to cover the cost of certain alternative healing techniques. The federal government has established an office whose entire focus is on alternative therapies. Most exciting of all is the influence of millions of new immigrants whose cultures integrate many aspects of natural medicine, spirituality and healing through touch. They have brought a greater awareness of the value of touch and healing to the general public.

When I co-authored my first book, *Massageworks,* in 1983, I was vice-president of the New York Chapter of the American Massage Therapy Association. Their national membership was about 4,000. Now it is over 30,000.

The growth of massage and bodywork as a profession has expanded beyond our wildest dreams and the quality of the work has also grown. Visionary teachers and healers have brought their massage, bodywork and healing skills to public view. The creation of On-Site Chair Massage has revolutionized bodywork by allowing people to get a 10-minute session with their clothes on.

This book, *Hands-On Healing,* is the next step. This is not simply a massage book; this is a book about transformation through touch. As you practice each of the 14 Hands-On Healing Techniques presented throughout these thirteen chapters you will learn how to give a great, relaxing massage, you will develop skills for eliminating aches and pains, and for creating and experiencing easy laughter, unembarrassed tears, a sense of spiritual expansiveness, philosophical independence and love. You will then be in touch with your deeper intuitive sensibilities.

I have learned that people who create what they want out of life have some basic characteristics in common. Among these are the ability to reduce stress and tension while overcoming fear, unproductive habits and other seemingly insurmountable obstacles. It is easier to achieve inner peace and contentment if you have access to the tools that will open the inner door. Hands-On Healing and Shaman Massage are just such tools. Life can be very demanding and complex. There seem to be obstacles to comfort, peace of mind and personal fulfillment around every corner. As you share Shaman Massage Techniques by practicing on family, friends, and loved ones you will begin to experience a personal transformation. You will find yourself defining what you are ready, willing and able to act upon in your life. How does this transformation come about?

Through the regular practice of the Hands-On Healing, Breathing, Vision Quests, Water Balancing, Shaman Massage, and Healing Through Movement Techniques in this book, you can find freedom from:

- Physical aches and pains
- Stress
- Tension
- A sense of aimlessness
- Spiritual Confusion
- Shyness
- Poor motivation
- Procrastination
- Lack of time management skills
- Lack of inspiration
- Lack of motivation
- Lack of clear goals and direction
- Poor priority planning skills
- Ineffective communication
- Lack of the skills necessary to create a support network
- Lack of mentors, friends or associates to advise you in times of stress
- A tendency to react to obstacles from fear rather than creatively responding to them

This book initiates you into what Gabrielle Roth, the Respected Urban Shaman and Dance Master, calls the five sacred powers natural and necessary for survival: the power of being, the power of loving, the power of knowing, the power of seeing, the power of healing. These are the real powers.

The book includes extensive drawings, photographs and charts that illustrate steps necessary to allow that transformation to take place without discipline, willpower or struggle.

The transformational steps in this book will give you a solid foundation. They are not pat answers or intimidating formulas. They are clear, concise, and are presented in a creative, enjoyable and easily followed step-by-step format that will make self-assessment and positive results a reality. Get ready for miracles through Hands-On Healing the Shaman's way.

CHAPTER 1

@

WHAT IS A HEALER?
WHAT IS A SHAMAN?

It isn't easy to define what a Shaman is and does. In most cultures, a Shaman is a healer whose power and knowledge derives from an intimate, ongoing relationship with personal angels, saints, guiding spirit or an inner voice. These inner contacts are unique in that they occur primarily, although not exclusively, while the Shaman is in a non-ordinary or "altered" state of consciousness. While in this state the Shaman takes an inner journey into the realm of the spirit and is given intuitive messages, guidance and instruction in inner wisdom and personal empowerment.

Traditionally Shamans lived in aboriginal, indigenous or native cultures. In Africa a Shaman or healer may be known as "sanoma" and "okomfo" if he is a prognosticator or diviner. If they are herb gatherers who create medicine blends from the fields and forests they may be known as "inyanga" and "dunseni." But there are many urban Shamans and individuals whose Shamanic practices integrate elements of many cultures. These are often known as Shamanic Practitioners. Most Shamans use various sacred tools to open themselves to an altered state of consciousness.

Many people are reluctant to study traditional Shamanism due to the belief that it will be at odds with their religious beliefs— that speaking to or being directed by nature spirits is a form of idolatry. Despite this reaction, many people have been drawn to Shamanism. This may be because the Shaman is a living example of the holistic philosophy that sees an interaction and relatedness between the physical, emotional and spiritual. The Shaman is the embodiment of holism. When mental health professionals evaluate

Shamans, they seem truly stumped. From an orthodox point of view, the Shaman may seem mentally ill, delusional, even insane. Shamans speak in ways and act out what they experience in ways that don't fit our rational, modern ways.

While hands-on healers may use Shamanic techniques, all healers are not Shamans, though in one way or another all Shamans are healers. If not healers of individuals, Shamans can be seen as healers for the community and even for the planet. Each culture may define a Shaman differently but there is one thing that all Shamans have in common. As defined in the original Siberian usage of the word, a Shaman is a type of spiritual healer found in tribal cultures. Shamanic practice seems to arise out of the basic human need for self-knowledge and divine knowledge, regardless of century, culture, climate, or geographical location.

Joseph Campbell, the respected anthropologist, defined the Shaman as "a person, male or female, who has an overwhelming psychological experience that turns him (or her) totally inward. The whole unconsciousness opens up and the Shaman falls into it."

As people develop a greater interest in alternative approaches to healing, especially in touch and massage, there has been a parallel growth of interest in native, Shamanic and aboriginal healing techniques. Within Native American, African and Latin American cultures we often hear of healers and medicine men (also known as Shamans) who can produce results unavailable to even the most sophisticated Western physician. We learn that many of the healing techniques now popular in our own culture (bodywork, massage, acupressure, movement reeducation, meditation, prayer, flower remedies, music, dance, and herbal oils) are key tools in Shamanic healing.

This chapter has a threefold purpose:

(1) to give you a better understanding of the history and development of Shamanic practice
(2) to open the door for you to engage your own healing potential
(3) to teach you the first two healing touch tools.

@ The Beginning

America is fast becoming a multicultural society. Many of our African, Asian and Latin American citizens have brought aspects of their healing and spiritual traditions with them. This phenomenon, combined with an increase of interest among anthropologists, theologians, health and medical researchers and students of natural healing, has brought Shamanic tradition to the public eye.

Using Joseph Campbell's definition it becomes quickly apparent that Shamans can be found throughout the world. There are Chinese, Irish, Latin American and African Shamans. There are Christian mystics and Jewish cabalists whose spiritual practices are in alignment with the definition of Shamanism.

What seems to link Shamans from various cultures is that they can enter realities not usually perceptible to people who are not able to enter an altered state of consciousness. Shamans are messengers in that they are capable of bringing back from these realities healing and helpful knowledge for themselves and others.

How does one enter a Shamanic state? Traditionally Shamanic states can be induced in many ways, the most common of which, in the West, is using monotonous sounds, such as steady drumming or chanting. How does the Shaman heal? By sourcing wisdom and spiritual knowledge from angels, spirit guides and saints whom the Shaman encounters while in an altered state of consciousness and sharing this knowledge with someone in need of healing. A Shaman needs knowledge of tools and techniques for entering an altered state of consciousness. When this altered state takes place the Shaman may experience a diminished sense of self, a shift or distortion in the perception of time, a reduction in inhibitions, and a decrease in the ability to discriminate between self and other objects and individuals. When in this altered state the Shaman can access realities that would normally be beyond the understanding of individuals whose consciousness is usually focused on the mundane aspects of daily life. The Shaman walks the thin line between "normal" reality and mystic knowledge. In an altered state, he can intentionally experience, as reality, those domains that ordinary people only experience in dreams and through mythology. There is a saying that life is not a series of lessons to be learned, but a series of messages to be heard. If one ignores the message, one doesn't learn the lesson. It is the role of the Shaman to retrieve vital messages for the healing of specific people, a small community, the larger community of man, or for the planet.

Many people assume that all herbalists or natural healers are also Shamans. This is not the case. What defines a Shaman is the means by which he sources information. Natural healers may have wonderful knowledge and great healing skill, but the Shaman obtains power from an alternative reality. Whether it comes from nature spirits, saints, channeling or from an inner voice contacted while in a deeply meditative state, the Shaman dips into a deep well and hears an inner voice.

In traditional native culture the Shaman may be told by guiding spirits to recommend common herbs that everyone in that culture is familiar with. In other cases the Shaman may recommend remedies that make no intellectual sense and yet create miraculous results. Decades ago an uneducated Christian man named Edgar Cayce would go into trance states and make unusual recommendations to cure conditions for people that he had not even met. He was so accurate, both in his diagnosis and treatment recommendations, that to this day people study these case histories through the Association of Research and Enlightenment, an organization formed to continue Edgar Cayce's work. Though certainly not a native Shaman in the traditional sense of the word, Edgar Cayce seemed, as is the case with many traditional Shamans, to journey into some realm or region of the spirit for his information. Native Shamans may do the same and even directly inquire of the plant spirits before recommending them as a remedy. Shamans may interpret dreams by speaking with dream spirits or even entering a dream to question forms that appear in that dream in order to share key information with the dreamer. No matter how a Shaman does his work, his wisdom and power is given to him through the spirits that have chosen to support him and help him on his mission.

The services offered by Shamans are uniquely based on the cultural setting. My own training focused on herbs, ceremonial work for transformational events, guidance through rites of passage, bringing my students together with their spirit helpers, and healing through touch.

There is no universal voice that speaks to each Shaman. The relationship between a Shaman and his spirit guides is a highly personal one. In some cultures, spirit guides can include devas, angels, gods and goddesses known only to that specific tribe. Some Shamans communicate with spirit guides that are known only to them and not to other members of their tribal group and culture. Shamans among indigenous peoples often speak to the spirits of plants and animals, rivers, mountains or even the five elements of ether, air, water, fire, and earth. Asian Shamans often speak with the spirits of deceased family members, ancestors or the ancestral spirits of other villagers.

While most anthropologists and students of Shamanism focus their studies on the traditional Shamanism of indigenous cultures, there is another type of Shamanic practice. This is often called Contemporary Shamanism or Core Shamanism.

◉ How Does One Become a Shaman?

There are three paths that people have taken to become Shamans in native cultures. These three paths are applicable today for the Western Shaman as well. These are:

1) an extreme emotional or life challenging event or crisis
2) Inner call—Shaman by birth
3) selection, initiation and guidance by a Sage, Master or elder

◉ Extreme Emotional or Life Challenging Event

The most intense means by which a person becomes aware of Shamanic destiny is through an emotional or life challenging event. This may be a minor realization or the equivalent experience to a sharp whack to the back of the head with a spiritual two-by-four. A chronic medical condition, the loss of a job, or the death of a loved one can cause a person to be emotionally or physically imprisoned for a long time, as can a degenerative disease, coma or physical handicap, deep emotional turmoil, or a near-death experience.

Events of this nature will tend to cause a radical shift in our sense of reality and our relationship with the external world. They lead to introspection and a realization that life is not a dress rehearsal, that the reality of our lives is in this very moment. Sometimes "this moment" is one of joy and celebration and sometimes it is great loss. When you begin to rethink the meaning of life, a transformation may take place in your sense of personal identity. When the ego self is assaulted or your sense of who you are is shattered, you may turn—in desperation, in surrender, in humility or simply in prayer—to the divine power within. We look for divine assistance. At that moment the spirit world calls and the Shamanic path is open to you. It is at this time that spirit guides, and angels come.

Traditionally, those Shamans who have been through the same experience or have a deep wisdom about such states can guide and support the individual through the event and interpret the spiritual message that such an event brings with it. The Shamanic Sages I studied with have always emphasized that "if you love you always have enough of what you need, and you are never given more than you can handle." Therefore, if you have love you also have faith and hope because, like love, faith and hope are free and unlimited. With love you always have what you need so long as you choose love instead of fear. When you are in a state of fear, it is doubtful that you will ever have what you need.

Living life is the same as being in a school. In any crisis there is a purpose and often that purpose is to send you a message. You are never sent a lesson that is beyond your understanding. You always reach your next step either smoothly and voluntarily, or by kicking, screaming and getting dragged there. It is the belief that you are given more than you can handle that creates the experience you are being dragged through with much emotional and spiritual struggle! The key is to create focus. The greater the intention, the greater the access to the inner voice.

Jason Shulman, a teacher of concepts relating to cabala and mystic Judaism, speaks of intention in this way. "Kavanah—the Hebrew word for intention—is often used to describe one of the most important qualities we need to bring to spiritual activity to make it effective. We have all had the experience of wanting, needing and focusing our will, yet often the thing we want to happen does not happen. Kavanah works because it is more than using our will and ability to focus: it also means "to make straight" and "to put right." And when we straighten the way by opening our heart to pure presence, we are lifted to a level where we can become aware of Creator-consciousness, not as myth or distant hope, but as the ongoing process of Creation in which we play a vital part. Being in Kavanah is being in a state of non-separation—an awakened state of intimacy with the world."

This is why many Shamans teach that crisis is a spiritual call and is a privilege as well. It is having the Shaman's guidance and support that makes the experience so important and worthwhile. It is the effort of the individual, combined with healing and guidance of the Shaman and the grace of the spirits, that brings the individual out from the other side. When the crisis has passed, and if the seeker accepts a Shaman's calling, then initiation takes place and a disciplined program begins under the guidance of the Sages and the helping spirits.

@ *Inner Call—Shamans by Birth*

Some individuals have a calling to a spiritual life even when they are children. This knowing may come in the form of dreams or from a feeling of harmony with nature; some feel connected to angels or nature spirits, while others wish to serve their family or community as a healer or "Sage."

@ *Selection by Elders*

There is a common saying that when the student is ready, the teacher appears. This is true. I met my own Shamanic teacher through dreams. In fact, I originally read a book by him. Not only did I not have an interest in it, but I was actually bored by it. Years later I began to have dreams of him. It was only after some correspondence and a series of mystical, intuitive events that I was initiated into this spiritual work. Years later I read a section of a wonderful book which was part of a large anthology. It was only later I realized it was the same book I had read years earlier and found to be boring! When you are selected by a Shaman or Sage it is because you are ready. When the student is ready the teacher appears.

@ *The Lure Beyond Ordinary Reality*

Some individuals feel a longing to exist in an extraordinary or non-ordinary spiritual reality. This pain of longing causes some people to feel that they are strangers in this world, as if this world is not their true home and yet they know they have work to do here. At some point the individual will be called to the work of being a Shaman or healer. A point eventually comes when the seeker either chooses to accept the calling or refuses to do so and chooses to lead an ordinary life.

However a person is drawn to this work, the seeker must act when the time is right, must respond out of a desire to serve and not out of ego satisfaction. Spirit guides have a different operating model than we do and must be able to surrender to the process while maintaining personal integrity and clarity.

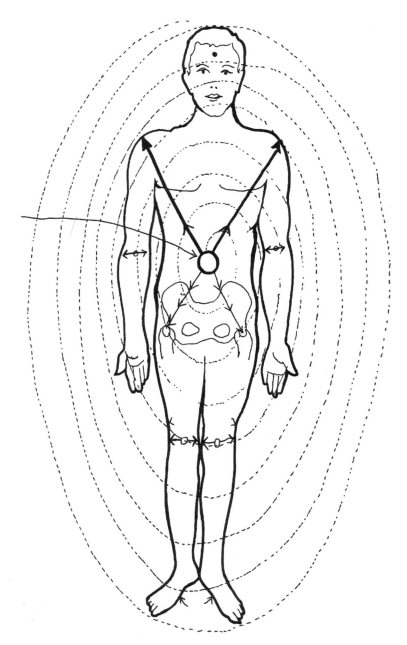

Chi Healing arises through the Vision Quest.

◉ Training

The relationship between a seeker and a Shaman or Sage is a uniquely personal process. Each seeker has a different destiny and different tools to offer in service. As such, the program for one seeker will be different than for another. In native cultures traditional Shamans may use many different tools—including fasting, meditation, dreaming, and asceticism, in combination with altered states of consciousness—to understand the role Shamanism will play for them. Some cultures may use physical isolation, and other more intensive processes to open the seeker's inner vision to their spirit guides. Traditional Shamans may use various ceremonial objects including masks, drums, rattles, musical instruments and costumes in their work. These may be used within the training process as well.

◉ The Vision Quest

A key element to Shaman practice is called the Vision Quest. It is the process of opening one's inner sense in order to hear the inner voice.

Lao Tsu, the great Chinese mystic, calls this inner voice the Tao. He describes this inner voice as the drop in the ocean. It is, in its primal form, both tranquil and pure. In the world it is knotted to the mind at the third eye Chakra and carried in the body. With all of the desires, emotions and sensory stimulation that makes the mind act the way it does, the Vision Quest draws the attention out of the worldly domain and into the spiritual domain. As storm clouds hide the stars, the storm clouds of the mind form a veil that temporarily hides the Shamanic voice from the person within whom it resides. As the storm clouds change their shape and form, making the stars appear and then disappear, so does the individual's spiritual focus waver from the spiritual domain to the world and back again. But in the end the North Star will guide the seafarer to his destination. So does the inner voice, through its sweetness to the inner taste and the light and sound it produces [which can only be heard with the inner senses] lead man to the Light. The Vision Quest is the means of beginning this journey.

For many Shamans the Vision Quest may begin with periods of solitude and quiet. Varying Shamanic traditions may associate solitude with long vigils into the night, fasting, extended periods of walking while guided by inner spirits (the Australian walkabout) ascetic practices (raw exposure to the weather) listening for inner light and sound, and meditation. As extreme as some of these practices sound, they are not always extreme for the Shaman. Since Shamanism is a response to an inner calling, the Vision Quest may actually come about through an intense response to this calling. The Vision Quest may bring about fundamental changes in how the Shamanic seeker views the physical and the spiritual worlds. More than just a simple change, often a great transformation takes place.

This tranformation can take many forms. My own process began with an emotional crisis in 1972. I had no vision and my life seemed aimless. I realized that up to that point of my life, I had been satisfied with physical pleasures and was unaware of the essence of my being. I had come to realize that there is more to life, but I didn't have a clue as to what is was. It was at this time that I met my first teacher, Vincent, and began the rite of passage which, under Vincent's guidance, became my Vision Quest. Though we speak about rites of passage in Western culture, it is seldom that these rites or transformations ever take place.

When a person has been through a rite of passage, one moves from childhood into adulthood; not just an adulthood defined by years, but by emotional and spiritual emergence. At this time a person without a vision or a mission will actively experience tremendous discomfort and aimlessness. One must understand that there is a difference between the content of experience that one wishes to have and the form in which it takes place. The content of experience can never be destroyed since it is not a physical thing. It is an internal process that is on a visceral, emotional level. Form can always be destroyed; that is why a person with a clear vision may be rich or poor but is deeply content with life, while the person who has wealth or great material possessions but does not have a clear sense of vision or mission, can be likened to a dog chasing its tail. Such a person spends all his time worrying about getting more or keeping what he has. A poor person who is attached to material form and has no vision is no better or no worse than a wealthy person in the same position. There is absolute spiritual, physical and emotional freedom for that person who has a clearly defined vision and an honest sense of who they are. The actual discrepancy between the vision and the self-assessment will create the fuel that moves that person forward in life, moment by moment, minute by minute, hour by hour, day by day, week by week, month by month, year by year.

Through a process of fasting, meditation and inner inquiry, I passed through the the process of self-involvement to the knowledge that I wanted to help others to self-knowledge and healing. In time, I began to see that much of this healing sensibility was going to be through my hands and through the touch application of hands-on healing.

Vision Quests are often made at what are called sacred places or power spots. These geographical locations are considered places where intense energetic concentration can be easily sensed and experienced. There are such places in Sedona, Arizona, Mount Shasta, California; and in the Catskill mountains in New York State. In was in the Catskills where my own Quest took place.

The study of these "spirit vortexes" is called geomancy. Such places are, in a sense, the Chakras of the earth. According to Nicholas R. Mann, the author of *Sedona: Sacred Earth*, "The art of geomancy has always been an integral part of architecture and landscape in China. There, the practice of Feng-Shui aimed for the achievement of terrestrial harmony through the balancing of the elements of the natural landscape."

◉ Use of Psychoactive Plants

Many seekers on the Shamanic path assume that the use of psychoactive substances (hallucinogenic drugs and plants) is an essential element in accessing altered states of consciousness. Much of this comes from reading the books of Carlos Castaneda and other early writers who introduced Shamanism to a wider audience. It is true that in many indigenous cultures visions, dream states and other consciousness shifts can be facilitated through hallucinogenic plants and other psychoactive substances, but this is not the only way. Simply "dropping acid" or doing "shrooms" (hallucinogenic mushrooms) does not make one a Shaman. Shamans within indigenous cultures have a deep understanding and respect for the spirits of plants and see these psychoactive agents as gifts from plants with a specific spiritual purpose. Getting access to this wisdom is not like buying instant chocolate pudding, mixing it up and eating it. It requires a long intense process with subtle guidance both within and without through elders or a mystic Sage.

In the early 1970s, when I began my own work, I expressed an

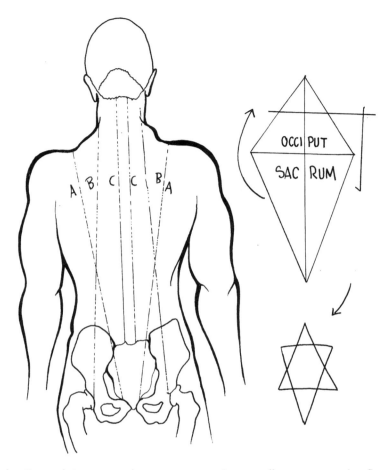

In the Sacred Anatomy there are esoteric as well as structural reflexes. The Occiput Triangle Resting on the Sacral Triangle are Sacred Symbols in ancient Egypt and in Mayan Culture. They also form the Christian Cross. If the Occipital Triangle sinks down and the Sacral Triangle Rises they form the Jewish Star of David.

early interest in psychoactive substances as a part of my Shamanic quest but on the direction of my teacher, Vincent, and subsequent teachers I never explored them.

@ Connecting to Your Own Shamanic Myths and Symbols

Within traditional Shamanism, a student would study tribal lore and symbols. This is a means for connecting to one's personal spirit guides. This process takes time, and part of the purpose of this book is to help you connect to this process with healing touch as the primary medium. Self-actualization is one of the doors that can be used to know and understand one's spirit guides and the power of the Shaman. Healing through touch, and storytelling, combined with music, and myths concerning my own cultural history, are the ways I have been given to tap into this power.

◉ Becoming a Practicing Shaman

If you are ready to follow the guidelines in this book and practice them, then you have stepped onto the Shaman's path. You do not require formal training, only the commitment to heal and be healed. It is the success you have in applying these principles that will open the Shaman's path to you. To practice on the Shaman's path is to expand your knowledge, wisdom, personal clarity and ability to serve and help others and nurture yourself.

◉ Healing the Spirit

The use and application of Shaman massage is an empowering process. When you are in a state of emotional or spiritual stress and anxiety, your personal power and life force are weak and out of balance. Shaman massage is a means for the restoration of this power. How? By defining where the energy imbalance lies and through song, dance, visualization and touch patching that "hole" or "gap" in a person's energy. It also involves the removal of any negative or disempowering thought patterns.

◉ Herbal Healing

In most indigenous cultures Shamans use herbs in many different ways. In Shaman massage herbs are used in three ways: 1. aroma therapy; 2. herbal baths; and 3. flower remedies.

◉ Bodywork

Many Shamans have skills in structural or energetic bodywork. The focus of this book is the application of these tools for your own healing and personal growth.

◉ Divination

Divination is a Shamanic technique for accessing information about something from "unseen" sources. Some Shamans look for

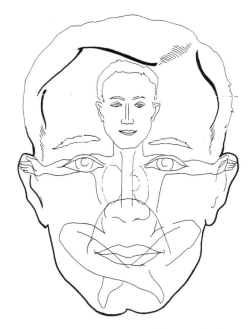

The Vision Quest to Self-Knowledge.

patterns in nature or use divining tools, such as stones, runes, sticks, or cards. Shamans may use divination tools, such as a pendulum and ask their spirit guides how to understand the information they impart. Some Shamans practice what is known as "channeling." In channeling the Shaman may become an open space for messages from their spirit guides or may even journey into the spirit world and inquire of the spirits for guidance or specific information.

@ Ceremony and Ritual

Shaman work is not rationalistic or intellectual in any sense. Shamans have an independent, Lone Ranger quality that causes them, without any seeming pattern, to do what they think is appropriate or what the inner voices direct them to do. Unlike a religious leader, a Shaman does not use a holy book or a list of prescribed standard rites and rituals. Shamans are rule breakers and rule makers. They are untraditional in every sense of the word, yet they are part of an ancient and deeply focused tradition. The world view that the Shaman lives in is as unconventional as the healing techniques a Shaman uses.

❦ The Shaman's World View

As different as each Shaman tradition may be, there are links of similarity among indigenous people throughout the world. One of these is the belief in a three-part structure of the cosmos. I refer to these as the three domains of spirit.

Each of these three domains is a fountain of understanding, power, and knowledge for the Shaman. In some cultures these three domains may be further divided into other realms and subdivisions in these realms. Some Shamans may have an internal connection with one realm but not the others and may visit or focus on personal power places only known to them. Most Shamans have a personal place, a hidden realm, a nameless reality where they go for their own guidance, rejuvenation, or healing.

❦ Sourcing Shamanic Power

In most cultures, Shamans understand that their work involves being focused within while detaching from the self. This may seem contradictory but it is not. In Shamanic work the Shaman is the bringer of messages, and in order to receive the message one must connect to specific helping spirits. These spirit guides may change as each spirit's need to work with a particular Shaman comes to an end.

In a sense it could be said that a Shaman's work is derived from grace and humility. It is a form of spiritual interdependence, for in the Shamanic relationship we are opening doors for miracles to happen. The Shaman is compassionate, humble and loving. Through service the Shaman contributes by making life better for others. These qualities bring the Shaman the service of the spirits.

A boastful, self-involved and egotistical Shaman will soon find himself working alone and without the guidance of the spirits that are essential to a Shaman's work.

There is no conflict between mainstream religion and spiritual experiences derived from Shamanic work. The experiences ascribed to various adepts, mystics, sages, Rebbes and saints directly mirror Shamanic work. It is likely that many great mystics, respected and praised in Christianity, Islam, Judaism, Hinduism and Buddhism, were themselves healing through touch.

The Shaman's path is not limited to any religious or spiritual tradition. It is a personal path involving a deep and intimate connection between helping spirits, spirit guides, and angels. It is an inner mystic journey that fills life with joy and contentment.

@ Core Shamanism

Shamans and Shamanic practitioners do not always come from particular indigenous cultures. Many live in cities and in modern society. Many Shamanic practices, massage techniques, myths, healing tools, and symbols are integrated and given a culturally neutral quality by Shamans around the world. Michael Harner, founder and director of the Foundation for Shamanic Studies, coined the term "Core Shamanism" to describe the practices of many modern practitioners. These techniques can be integrated into virtually any religious tradition in any culture.

One of the key techniques associated with Shamanism is the shifting of consciousness from an ordinary state to a Shamanic state. It is not easy to explain what this state is other than to say that it is similar to what one might experience in dreams or myths. The distinction lies in the fact that when we are embraced in myths and dreams we are usually unconscious, but the Shamanic state is very conscious. It is simply an extraordinary state of consciousness.

@ Shamanism Is a Practical Experience

Shamanic massage is an excellent tool for personal spiritual growth. The visualization and breathing techniques applied with Shaman massage will help you focus attention on the positive aspects of your daily life. When applying or receiving Shamanic massage there is an awakening of a subtle, hidden knowledge of self. It is as if you are getting in touch with a hidden forgotten wisdom. Through music and drumming you will contact an inner place that you were not aware of. Shamanic massage, and the awakening techniques used with it, create a link to an ancient wisdom.

The discovery of the Shamanic path will create a sense of meaning that may lead a person to a deeper sense of his own religious upbringing or open the door to an entirely new spiritual experience.

If Shamanism is an unusual or extraordinary concept to you, you may soon be surprised to know that from childhood through adulthood there are many events and experiences in our lives that are Shamanic in nature. A person who experiences déjà vu, feels an inner call to a spiritual path, or experiences a "state of flow" during the artistic or creative process, is having an experience associated with a Shamanic state. Often in our homes we have a favorite "power spot," certain foods that we connect to, certain songs, chants or pictures that affect us on a deeply emotional level. Some of these things may even mesmerize us. There is a natural mystic quality to all of us and we are often sensitive to those things that maximize or magnify these qualities.

@ Teachers

One cannot become a Shaman or a Shamanic practitioner just by reading books, listening to audio tapes or viewing films and videos. Ultimately one must meet a Shaman who is willing to accept an apprentice. Teachers in non-ordinary reality come in many different forms and in many different cultures. The Shamanic student may acquire the required knowledge through regular journeys into the spirit world through the guidance of the Shamanic teacher. In the end this training will support the student in achieving the skills necessary to become an effective practitioner.

@ Life Experiences

When a Shaman student is working with an indigenous elder, or teacher, he will be guided by this teacher through an initiation that will include a sequence of visionary experiences that will open the door of the spirit world. These experiences may include long periods of chanting, dancing, fasting, meditation, solitude, dream work, intuitive exercises.

In my early studies, my teacher, Vincent, would have us fast on water anywhere from 3 to 40 days as both a physical and spiritual cleansing. Many teachers use psychotropic plants for visionary experiences. My teacher always frowned upon this practice outside of aboriginal Shamanic settings. He felt that the use of plants in this way was irresponsible without years of intense study, training, and supervision under a Shaman. The irresponsible use of hallucinogenic plants can be dangerous for Western participants, and since they are illegal in the United States, I do not recommend using these tools.

@ *Becoming a Shamanic Practitioner*

If you were being trained by a native Shaman or an elder, they would let you know when you were competent to work with others. This book cannot, of course, replace a teacher. Knowing how to apply the techniques of Hands-On Healing cannot make you a competent Shamanic practitioner any more than a college degree makes you an expert in your chosen field.

By consistently practicing the bodywork, visualizations, herbal and other tools described in this book, you will develop confidence, humility, clarity, sensitivity and skill in Shamanic practices. Only your own honesty and clarity concerning your healing gifts will define what you have achieved.

The key to my work has been the balancing of the Western rational approach to consciousness with the cultivating of my own sensitivity. In this process I have attempted to gain a deeper respect for the river of life-energy within everything.

Modern science is beginning to verify that everything in the universe carries a particular vibration. Neuroscientists, physicists, anesthesiologists, philosophers and researchers of virtually every specialty are exploring consciousness. Studies have included research on the brain wave patterns of meditating monks, the abilities of certain Yogis to control voluntarily what were thought to be involuntary body functions, high-tech brain imaging research, and thought experiments.

Over 34 scholarly books on consciousness were published between 1991 and 1997, and two scientific journals on consciousness have been started in recent years. In the scientific study of Shamanism and consciousness there is not only a focus on answering key questions but also on the dilemma of discovering what are the key questions. We must learn how to discuss the questions and answers in a way that will give us a greater understanding of consciousness and Shamanism and how these influence, health, well-being and spiritual development from a multicultural perspective. The difficulty of all these studies is that the intellectual vocabulary required to present a unifying principle for all the theories on consciousness, or even to discuss Shamanism and consciousness, doesn't really exist to this day. It is in its infancy. In fact many scientists and researchers believe that modern science, as it presently exists, is incapable of developing a language to address the intricacies of the conscious mind and altered states of consciousness.

◉ What Is the Energy Body?

Among healers and Shamans, the energy body is also called the etheric body. Webster defines etheric as: "Coming from the word ether, that which fills the upper nature of space, or Heaven—a medium, that in the undulatory theory of light, permeates all space, transmitting transverse waves of energy." From this definition, we may see that Shamanic massage is *light work,* and that the energy body is vibrational in nature. Shamanic healers offer a touch without touch. They somehow influence an invisible energy flow that surrounds the physical form. Some healers can see this energy field with its luminous colors and its radiant glow. The energy body merges with the physical body through the Chakras. This balances the etheric field, which defines the quality of physical being more than any other factor.

◉ The Practical Applications of Energy Healing

Energy healing can take place through numerous techniques. A wonderful approach to begin with is the polarity self-help exercises and manipulations developed by Dr. Randolph Stone. Dr. Stone recognized that Westerners are usually too busy or too lazy to devote long periods of time to exercise. Thus he designed a highly effective series of "easy stretching postures" which use 15 minutes of daily movement and sound to give you feedback on what's happening with the energy in your body. I have integrated these exercises with dance movements, strength building and hatha Yoga.

The Shamanic healing touch and massage techniques include all types of touching and pressure, ranging from deep tissue movement to light etheric contacts. The energies in the body have qualities that can be understood in terms of the natural elements: ether, air, fire, water, and earth. When touch and the five elements come together, you have energy healing.

The most important aspect of Shaman massage is that it helps create mental awareness and emotional mastery. Part of the beauty of Shaman massage is its inherent creative possibilities. Once the

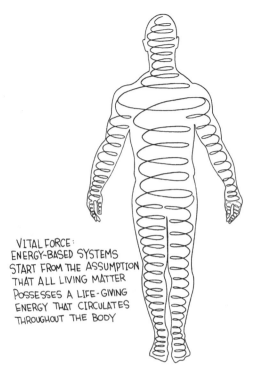

VITAL FORCE:
ENERGY-BASED SYSTEMS
START FROM THE ASSUMPTION
THAT ALL LIVING MATTER
POSSESSES A LIFE-GIVING
ENERGY THAT CIRCULATES
THROUGHOUT THE BODY

The Energy Body: There is a life-giving and healing energy that flows throughout the body but cannot be seen with the eyes.

respect for the energy has been established, it opens the door to the healing process taking place on all levels: emotional, structural, physical and spiritual. Shaman massage is an external symbol of an internal process. Your commitment to your own evolution determines whether or not Shaman massage will have only a short-term or a lasting transformative benefit. As you use the techniques presented throughout the book you will begin to acknowledge the magnificence of the energy within. The healing is in your hands. The key thing is to always listen to your intuition. It has consciousness; give it its due. Do the work as though the outcome depends on the elegance of your skill and realize that in actuality, the results depend on the energy, not you.

@ *Adapting Shamanism to Western Belief Systems*

In general, Shamanic practitioners subscribe to the three-part cosmology of traditional Shamans: the spirit world consists of upper, lower, and middle regions.

In Shamanism, there is no separation in the idea of man and nature: man is part of nature but is unconscious of where the connection lies. In the native tradition nature is sacred and there is no way to separate the minute aspects of our daily lives from the nature of spirit experience. In the Shamanic experience you do not feel separate from the creator. Rather you begin to see the creator in all things both living and the seemingly inanimate. The Taoist Shamans of China call this the ''10,000 things.'' The Divine Spirit is everywhere.

You may engage in fasting because it alters your consciousness, making you more aware of spiritual activity within you, the presence of spirits around you, or the spiritual insights that can arise in an altered state of consciousness. You might also fast for non-spiritual reasons, such as for physical health.

Achieving the altered state of consciousness may also involve sweat lodges, dance, music, pilgrimages, night vigils, vision quests, singing, chanting, staring at mandalas or many other practices individually or in combination. Many Shamanic practitioners incorporate Shamanic practices into their daily lives.

Many researchers believe that the entering of an individual into a Shamanic consciousness can be measured by when the person enters ''alpha state.'' This is a brain wave pattern measurable when people are involved with various events including deep prayer, meditation, biofeedback, and Shamanic drumming.

The fact that these patterns can be measured supports the concept that Shamanism is not something you can convey through words but an experience that can be duplicated through special training and consistent practice.

@ *Health and Healing*

In many native cultures the traditional Shaman's view is that one is afflicted with disease because there has been a loss of spiritual power. This may translate as an imbalance in the life energy or Chi. The balancing of Chi does not require the rejection of Western medicine but Western medicine cannot do the job alone, since there must be an integration of body, mind, and spirit for true healing to take place.

Many people who have been cured of a disease may exhibit emotional stress, guilt, shame, and fear of relapse. Shamanic tools, by addressing spiritual as well as emotional and physical needs, can create a balance that is beyond the capabilities of Western medicine. Shamanic practitioners can use touch, music, dance, the breath, visualization and a host of other ancient rituals to transcend our limitations and open us up to new possibilities.

The sacred rituals you may choose to utilize as a Shamanic practitioner can be rooted in your own religious background. Sacred music, Sufi dance, chanting, intense prayer or prayer beads are all useful.

Within African and Latin American spiritual practices there is often a thread of Shamanic sensibility that was lost in European-based practices, but this has begun to change. Many Americans of European descent are exploring Norse, Celtic, Saxon, cabalistic, Mediterranean, and mystic Christian rituals and practices that are clearly Shamanic in orientation. These rituals and ceremonies are being investigated, revived, and integrated into various healing and consciousness-raising systems. In a sense we are entering the millennium with the guidance of ancient wisdom.

The ability to heal is a gift. One should be humble and gracious in being able to access this energy. To heal is to act in partnership with the obvious and subtle energetic qualities that exist in every nook and cranny of the earth, whether the intellect is guiding you or angels and nature spirits.

Shamanic devices, whether musical instruments, dance, aromatic oils, or energy healing can serve as a carrier that transports the practitioner into other psychic domains. Past life memories and internal untapped wisdom come to the surface on a reality that is clearer and finer than the ordinary reality that was part of daily life before. The wants of the mind and the needs of the spirit become clear and concise as they merge as one.

It may take years of inner work and Shamanic practice to hear the inner spirit voices, but in the process of journeying, rediscovery takes place. Shamanic elders teach that there is a genuineness in all of us that stays hidden under a veneer of respectability and normalcy. Once you allow your inner voices to rise to the surface, you can live fully.

@ Tradition

A key element in the Shamanic process is your ability to reconnect with the earth. In Taoism this is seen as returning to the rhythm of Natural Law. This is something we possess as young children, but lose as we get older and become more socialized and influenced by external culture. Most Shamans have either a personal or cultural tradition that they use as a vehicle for reconnecting. I, for example, make great use of Klesmer music, a secular combination of Eastern European Jewish music with religious overtones and a strong influence of everything from Gypsy music to American jazz.

The essence of all Shamanic healing is love. Because Shamanic healing helps others to become whole, it is among the most powerful of tools for those whose "wholeness" had been taken from them. Shamans speak of "soul loss" as if a psychic portion of the soul has been removed or has left. The person still lives but is in a sense the "walking dead." This sense of lost self is often experienced by those individuals who have suffered through an ungrieved death, divorce, physical torture, rape, sexual abuse, divorce, a life challenging medical crisis, childhood abuse, physical trauma, emotional trauma, mental illness and addiction.

According to some scholars this soul loss is one of the ways that a person survives an exceedingly painful experience. The Shamanic practitioner is trained to connect to that part of the person's soul that has "left" and gently, lovingly bring it home to wholeness.

@ Shamanism and Healing

In the Shamanic view of health and sickness, disease results when a person turns away from the spiritual center. It is not to say that there are not genetic factors in health and disease. Rather it is the recognition that when one is in alignment with natural law (i.e. spirit power) the life force is strong and integrated. The illness moves into a "break" in the person's Chi, or life force. In the place of powerful, balanced energy a distorted unbalanced energy arises. The healing tools that are given life through body, mind and spirit recreate the environment where balanced "Chi" can flow.

The healer enters a Shamanic state of consciousness, calling upon angels, devas and other helping spirits and guides, then locates the blockage or distortion through inner voices, intuition, and the feeling for various pulses, heat or tingling in the hands.

When an imbalance is removed, it is neutralized through chants, ritualized baths, prayer, the burning of sage and other herbs and through the healing of touch.

Shamans have a sense of the emotions, the physical and spiritual. They are able to weave a harmonious connection between all of these human elements. In the end peace, serenity, harmony, love and contentment heal the ailing body and soul. Shamans have a spiritual sensibility that integrates the practical and the mystical and yet they are detached from the process. They are messengers who remain detached from the message.

As the great Chinese Sage Lao Tsu says in his 81-paragraph poem the *Tao Te Ching:*

> Therefore the sage manages affairs without action (wu-wei) and practises the teaching that uses no words (conveys instructions without the use of speech).

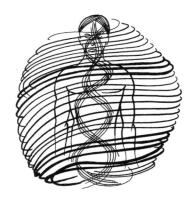

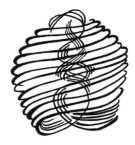

The Merging of the Emotional, Physical and Spiritual Bodies.

All beings emerge from the Tao yet it claims no authority;
He gives them life yet claims no possession;
He acts, but does not rely on his own ability.
He accomplishes his task, and yet he is detached from the results.
It is precisely because he does not claim credit that his accomplishment remains with him.

Shamanic healing is not limited to physical problems. It is enlivening, energizing, and spiritually uplifting. Through the clarity of the Shaman's inner vision a person comes to understand how the many aspects of life are interconnected. The results from Shamanic healing may be subtle and not always obvious. At other times results may be unexpectedly dramatic and mystical. Sometimes the process is like surfing a wave, but more often, the healing occurs gradually and in combination with other approaches, including herbs and massage.

When someone experiences a calling to Shamanic work it is easy to get trapped in clichés of spirituality and false humility, what the great Buddhist teacher Chogyam Trungpa Rinpoche called "spiritual materialism." Whether the calling is through an inner vision, a dream or an intellectual choice, the decision to enter Shamanic work is defined by the calling to do service for others and make a difference in the world. The spirits are guiding you; when you are called to enter this work, it will be made known to you.

One of the greatest messages I have ever received in my own Shamanic path was the information that at the moment you are ready, willing and able to act on a vision or calling, it takes place spontaneously without discipline or willpower. This concept is difficult for many people to understand because so many theories about success tell us that achievement is the end result of a long uphill battle in a hostile world. The truth is that we are always doing something at every second and the things that we are most ready, willing and able to do, we do without thought. It is an effortless process. When you are hungry you are ready, willing and able to eat. Breathing or awakening from a long sleep are things that simply happen. When it is time for something, it is time and it happens because it can do nothing else but happen. It is important that a person who is committed to service, Hands-On Healing or simply living a joyous and struggle-free life take a few moments every morning and explore those things that are important to them. With this introspection comes the desire to do those things that will create a desired result and which can be done as easily as taking a deep full breath.

I have learned that life is not a series of experiences or lessons to be learned. Through my Shamanic work I came to understand how pointless it is to see things as good or bad; it is really only effective to do this concerning moral issues. When we look back at our lives we can all see things that seemed positive which later turned out to be disasters and other things which, though appearing negative at the time, turned out to be great gifts. It is seldom that we can clearly see the long-term benefits or potential damage inherent in a particular event at a particular time. Therefore, it is important to understand that when your foundation is love and respect, everything that happens in your life is a gift. One of the stories that I was told by one of my mentors is that life is like a rosebush. The rose petals are beautiful to look at and they smell sweet. And, in order for a rose to be a rose it must grow on a thorny bush. See yourself as a beautiful silk cloth that has been placed on a thorny rosebush. It is your job to remove yourself from the bush, thorn by thorn. The more carefully and gently this is done, the less damage occurs to the cloth. This is the essence of doing things that you are ready, willing and able to do while being in the world but not of the world. It is the way to make effective choices without the need to make excuses. It is the path to understanding what a struggle-free life looks like. It is the path of the Shaman.

My experience over the last 25 years has shown me that all people have the potential for Shamanic vision and practice. By entering that path one can experience a greater sense of self and an immediate ability to positively impact the lives of others and the planet as a whole.

AN INTRODUCTION TO HANDS-ON HEALING AND SHAMAN MASSAGE TECHNIQUES

@ Energy Sourcing

This is the basic technique used to develop sensitivity to Chi. It is an essential skill for all energy-based healing and Shamanic work.

◎ Muscle Kneading

The Muscle Kneading Technique may be done across the muscle to break down superficial adhesions or simply to reduce muscle cramping and increase muscle tone and circulation.

◎ Polarity Similars

Polarity Similars is an extremely gentle technique. It is based on the concept that there is an energetic reflex action between certain body parts. By placing one hand on the point of blockage and the second on its corresponding reflex, the body's healing power is stimulated and the energy is balanced. There are hundreds of such reflex points. For simplicity and clarity, many of these reflex points are listed throughout the book.

◎ Chi Balancing

Chi Balancing is a technique for tapping directly into the body's healing energy field. It is a very gentle contact; at times the practitioner is barely touching the client or not touching them at all. It is one of the entry level techniques for those interested in becoming Shamanic practitioners.

◎ Rhythmic Pressure Point Massage

Pressure Point Massage is a Shamanic approach to what is commonly called acupressure. This approach can be applied in a number of ways:

1. Jin Shin: A pattern of prolonged holding (one to five minutes) of key acupressure points along the meridians.
2. "First Aid": This approach is less concerned with balancing energy and focuses more as an instant approach to pain and discomfort. Specific points are pressed for the temporary relief of common problems.

◎ Circular Pressure Point Massage

In addition to pinpointing energy blockages, this specialized form of Pressure Point Massage is used to relieve deep-rooted muscle tension, structural problems and restrictions in the range of motion. A rhythmic circular motion is the technique to choose for muscle spasms or cramps and is one of the main techniques for healing damaged tissue and reducing the formation of scar tissue after surgery or sprains. It can be done very lightly or with firm pressure.

@ Increasing Joint Motion

This is a gentle movement to help evaluate areas requiring healing and to improve flexibility in the joints. You can evaluate certain factors in a person's emotional life by the condition of the muscles associated with each joint. By working each joint through its range of motion you can release emotional holding points while reducing muscular tension.

@ Pull and Stretch Traction

This technique helps to expand tight muscles and restricted joints. A natural, non-stress traction it gives the person receiving it a sensation of openness and warmth throughout the body.

@ The Muscle Hug

This technique is used when a muscle is tight, flaccid, or weak. It is also valuable for those who are uncomfortable with deep kneading or any type of forceful massage. It is a gentle, effective technique.

@ Gravity Rocking

This very gentle technique is used to release surface tension and superficial energy blocks in the body and to stimulate the sensory motor nerves, thus readying the body for other techniques. Muscle Rock is excellent for removing both emotional and physical tension and consequently is a very good way to prepare the body for a complete Shaman Massage session.

Gravity Rocking is a very soothing technique that seems to create a sense of tranquility between the giver and the receiver in much the same way that a mother's rocking has a soothing effect on both the mother and baby. It is valuable for those in a state of fear or terror.

@ Expanding the Internal Chi

This is a passive preparation technique that is done prior to a full Hand-On Healing and Shaman Massage Session.

@ *Chakra Balancing*

Chakras are subtle "life fields" vibrating at specific frequencies and dynamically shifting in subtle sounds, shapes, and colors. Chakra balancing involves light touch on the body's energy centers especially those that energize Chi. Balanced Chakras are a key element in certain types of Shamanic practice.

@ *Connective Tissue De-armoring*

This is a combination of deep Transverse Muscle Kneading and Pressure Point Massage used to loosen and open the fascia. It is used to free emotional trauma from the system.

@ *Skin Rolling*

This is a powerful technique for freeing up emotional trauma. Among Mongolian Shamans it is a common belief that muscles "remember" early fears, traumas and painful experiences. These traumas are freed by lifting the skin and placing it between your thumb and your index and middle finger. It is then rolled in long, vertical strokes.

BASIC, INTERMEDIATE AND ADVANCED HANDS-ON HEALING AND SHAMAN MASSAGE TECHNIQUES.

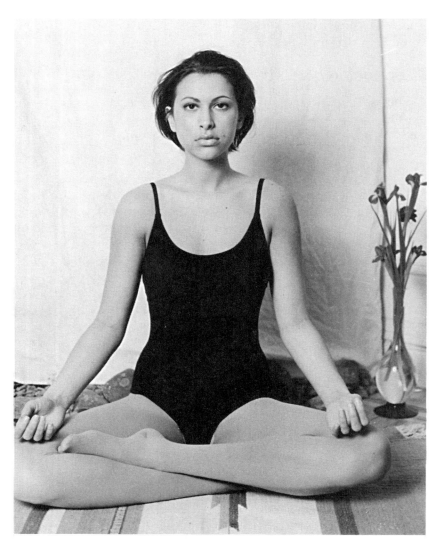

Energy Sourcing Position
(used with deep abdominal breathing).

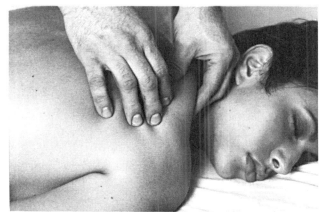

Muscle Kneading (muscle kneading on shoulder).

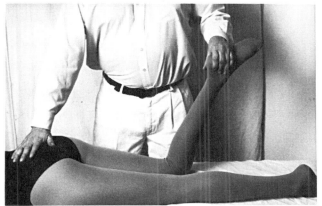

Polarity Similars (sacrum to heel).

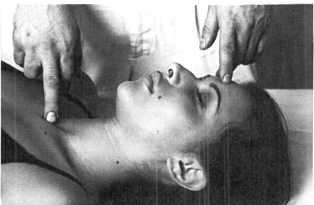

Chi Balancing (third eye and crest of sternum).

General Pressure
Point Massage
(Includes Circular
and Rhythmic
Techniques).

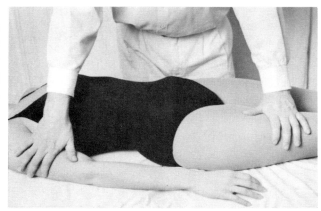

Increasing Joint
Motion (Back
Knee bend).

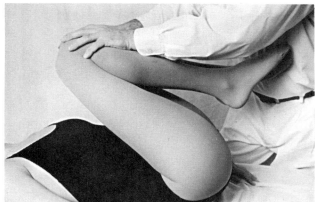

Pull and Stretch
Traction (to legs).

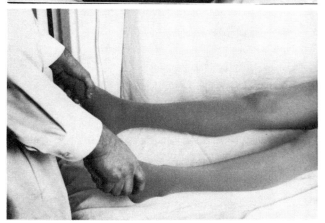

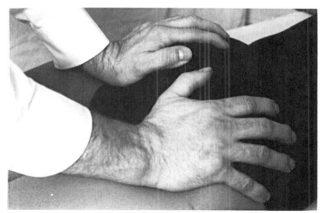

Muscle Hug (on buttocks).

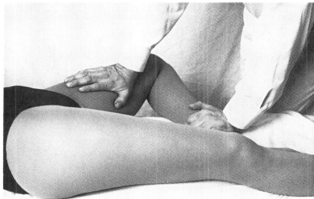

Gravity Rock.

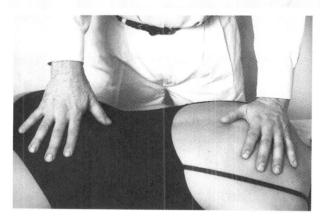

Chakra Balancing.

Connective
Tissue
De-armoring.

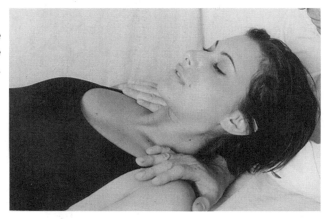

Skin Rolling
(shoulder blade).

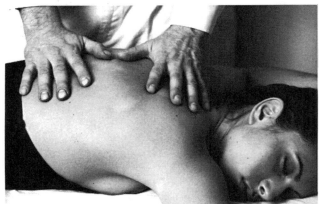

CHAPTER 2

@

MANY HEALERS, MANY PATHS

Healing through massage and energizing touch is a means for expressing the "power" that comes from the Shaman's internal connection to angels, helping spirits and natural law. This power is synonymous with the life force, Chi, logos, Tao, or divine energy that fills the universe. In almost all cultures Shamans have used the concentrated power of certain locations, people, rituals and objects. These power objects can include any number of forms. In my own work, aromatic oils, flower essences, crystals, stones have a spiritual meaning and importance. I use these objects in preparation for my healing massage sessions and to support me in maintaining my spiritual focus during these sessions.

@ The Way Touch Heals

Generally speaking touch heals in one of two ways: 1) structurally and 2) energetically.

@ Structural Healing

Therapeutic massage and traditional Swedish massage are the most common forms of structured massage. When mainstream physicians and academic publications inquire about massage and its effect on pathophysiology, this is the type they are generally drawn to. This is not surprising since in its scope and philosophical foundations, structural massage is the most Western and rational of the various types of touch. In order to be effective in the application of structural massage the practitioner must have an understanding of body mechanics, posture, pathology, anatomy and physiology, especially the names and key parts of the muscles, bones and nerves. Structured massage practitioners who also have an interest in the connection between chronic structural problems and psychological factors require specialized training in what is commonly called psychotherapeutic bodywork.

@ Benefits of Structured Massage

- Improvement of body alignment
- Increased circulation
- Pain reduction
- Increased sensory awareness
- Reduced stress
- Increased flexibility of the joints

Note: As you begin to practice structured massage techniques it is easy to become so focused on the details and specifics of technique that compassion and intuition get lost in the process. Always balance knowledge of the body with expression of the heart through compassion.

@ Energetic Healing

Virtually all Shamanic systems work with what Dr. Randolph Stone calls "The Wireless Anatomy." This is that part of us that exists prior to, through and around all the other anatomical systems. It underlies and supports the nervous system and the circulatory system and can be addressed through touch, visualization, homeopathic remedies, the inserting of needles into specific points and even through inhaling aromatic oils or pressing on specific reflexes on the body. The life force that exists in each of us, "The Wireless Anatomy" known as Chi, Ki, Prana and Qi, is the source of all healing. Energetic healing does not require hands-on contact. It works totally on a vibrational or energy level, as opposed to a structural level, and its purpose is to release the body's own self-healing energy wherever it may be blocked.

@ Benefits of Energetic Healing

- Greater sense of spiritual awareness
- Increased self-esteem

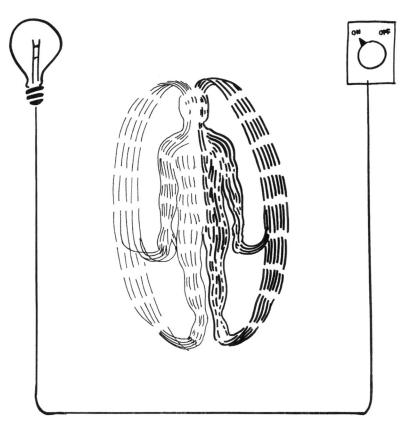

Healing with Energy. If electricity in your home is shorted out, the lights won't go on. If the Chi "life force" within your body is "shorted out," the power to coordinate movement, heal and function effectively physically, emotionally and spiritually, can't take place.

- Brings inspiration and motivation to consciousness
- Increased sensory awareness
- Reduced stress
- Reduced pain
- Increases healing of fractures, or broken bones and all injuries in which movement or manipulation of the joint is not recommended

Note: This technique is used when a person is so sensitive to touch that virtually any massage technique would create pain or discomfort. It is also wonderful for those under great emotional stress.

@ *Tools for Healing Touch*

Touch is the first response we have when we need to heal. What do you do when you bang your head? You rub it. Healing touch is a key element to achieving and keeping good health. If you are not being touched, hugged or massaged on a regular basis, you are doing yourself a great disservice. But what is the best technique? There are many, and before you learn Shamanic Massage, it is of great value to understand some of the more popular bodywork, massage and Hands-On Healing techniques that are available.

Alexander Technique: The Alexander Technique was created by a young Australian actor named Frederick Matthias Alexander. In the 1880s he lost his voice one night on stage. He saw numerous doctors for the problem, but found that whatever medications or other approaches prescribed for him were useless. He retired from the theater and spent the next ten years looking at the way he used his body when speaking and acting. He noticed that he had a habit of pulling his head back and down involuntary when he opened his mouth to speak.

Dozens of other small involuntary movements were part of a pattern that included lifting his chest and hollowing his back. To correct each of these movements, he worked in front of a mirror for ten years. He created the Alexander technique so he could help others learn to be more effective and careful when using their bodies.

Amma: A distant cousin of Shiatsu, it works both to free up energy blockages and to release tension in the muscles in the skin that results from congestion in the circulatory system, especially stagnant blood. Many believe that Swedish massage is the grandchild of Amma.

Bioenergetic Therapy: Developed by Alexander Lowen, M.D., and John C. Pierrakos, M.D., this work, heavily influenced by Wilhelm Reich, includes both manipulative procedures and special exercises designed to help a person get in touch with his/her tensions and release them through appropriate movement. Bioenergetic Therapy utilizes the body/mind system to help resolve emotional problems. Massage, controlled pressure, and gentle touching are used to relax contracted muscles.

Chua K'a*: This term means to sculpture out. It is an ancient Mongolian manipulation system. The technique consists primarily of a rolling of the skin in long, vertical strokes as well as deep manipulation of muscle and bone. The technique involves a process where emotional tension and associated traumas are released thus clearing the way for positive emotions.

Cranial-Sacral Balancing: The cranial-sacral system is the environment in which the brain and spinal cord function. Correcting imbalance here improves the functioning of the nervous system, thus reducing stress and enhancing the function and health of the whole body. Cranial-Sacral bodywork and energy healing is a gentle and effective method for evaluating and correcting imbalance and restriction throughout the body. A master Cranial-Sacral practitioner should be able to identify the subtle movements of the cranial bones and sacrum with palpation and demonstrate the specific techniques and protocols to evaluate and correct craniosacral dysfunction. Emotional trauma and repressed anger can lead to energetic imbalances throughout the system. This trauma often influences body rhythms that connect to reflexes of the cranial bones and down to the sacral bone at the base of the spine. On a structural level, the connective tissue inside the mouth may reflect stress in the cranial bones that can influence structure and function in the body. It is a step-by-step process that includes pain and disorders of the neck and imbalances in the skull. The masseter and buccinator muscles may be tight from years of clenching in anger or withholding tears.

The cranial bones that make up the skull are covered with a thick layer of connective tissue. This connective tissue goes down the temple and inside the jaw, splitting off into the layers of deep and superficial fascia of the neck and down into the trunk. When fascia and the associated muscles are imbalanced there is a chain reaction through the muscles in the mouth and face ending with a pulling effect on the vertebrae of the neck. This creates abnormal strain on the sphenoid bone and through the cranium. This reflects down to the hips and the sacrum. Many practitioners, among them

*Chua K'a is a service mark of Arica Institute, Inc. © 1973 Arica Institutes, Inc.

Dr. John Upledger and Franklin Sills have discovered simple systems for holding or balancing the rhythm of the cranial bones. It is subtle and highly effective work.

Do-in: This is an energy-based self-massage technique. Many of the techniques are similar to those found in Shiatsu; however, most of the Do-in points are located on the cranium, face, neck, and feet. Do-in is especially helpful in alleviating mental stress, tension headaches, and emotional fatigue.

Feldenkrais Movement: Moshe Feldenkrais, who developed this system, was a visionary Israeli physicist. Each action performed in the Feldenkrais method is composed of four major components— movement, sensation, feeling, and thought. Optimal functioning requires a balance of all four. As we leave childhood, our actions tend to be more and more governed by societal pressures, organization, and "accepted" images. These factors limit the development of our full potential and foster the growth of set patterns of thought, action and feeling.

In order to change the way we act, we must change our self-image and the motivations tied to it. Dr. Feldenkrais believed that awareness of our actions is the key to overcoming habitual patterns of thought and action and expanding our capabilities. Movement is the ideal medium in which to effect changes and is directly tied to the nervous system.

Healing the Emotions: Each one of us has feelings. We express our passions and sensibilities. We experience love and hate and an entire array of emotions. Our ability to be in touch with and express our emotions has a large part to play in the types of choices we make. Touch is among the most powerful tools for creating this emotional connection. The breath, visualization and aromatherapy can increase the effectiveness of the massage.

In my massage and aromatherapy model I have tended to work with the four basic emotions that many psychologists believe people are capable of experiencing. These emotions may be viewed differently from culture to culture.

Jin Shin Do: Combines gentle yet deep finger pressure on acupoints to release the tensions that stem from blockages along the body's energy channels.

Kahuna: This is a Polynesian-based energy healing system commonly practiced in Hawaii and the Philippines. It is similar in appearance to faith healing though it is different in concept. It is, in a sense, the "laying on of hands." This description, however, is really inadequate. In comparing Kahuna conceptually to other systems it is probably closest to Shiatsu or Amma. Philippine Kahuna practitioners may use the balls of their feet instead of their hands.

Muscular Therapy: Created by Ben Benjamin, Ph.D., a dancer and student of movement theory, it integrates massage and education in movement. Included in this system are deep massage treatments, postural alignment, reeducation in movement, and tension release exercises. Much of the movement work draws its philosophy from the writings of Mable Todd, Lulu Sweigard and Irmgard Bartinieff, each of whom helped foster a greater understanding of body mechanics and energy function. Muscular therapy has its strongest value in pinpointing the effects of misalignment caused by improper use of the body in relation to gravity and in recognizing the effects of emotional repression in causing postural problems. By reducing tension, Muscular therapy attempts to keep the body aligned, relaxed and healthy.

Myotherapy: This is a system of acupressure using fingers, knuckles, and elbows on specific trigger points. Unlike Shiatsu, this system, developed by the late Bonnie Prudden, focuses on relieving muscle spasm and pain, rather than the energy pathways that are the specialty of Asian and Shamanic healing systems.

Naprapathy: Developed by Oakley Smith DC. in the early part of this century, Naprapathy is a gentle, non-force system of spinal and joint manipulation. It is unique in that it uses a system of charts and symbols by which the practitioner can record the location and severity of body tension and soreness as well as the specific manipulations needed to correct the problem. In a Naprapathic session, the practitioner will gently push and probe with the hands to test for resistance in the soft connective tissue. All Naprapathic schools in the United States are in Illinois; consequently that is where most Naprapathic practitioners are located. There is also a school in Stockholm, Sweden. Naprapathy is directed primarily on the ligaments encasing the spinal column. Connective tissue in this area intimately affects the functioning of the spinal nerves.

Polarity Therapy: More a healing system rather than a massage or bodywork technique, this approach was synthesized by Randolph Stone DC, DO, ND, and is a combination of five-element theory, Western physics, Chakra balancing, structural and energy-based bodywork and aspects of nutritional, herbal and emotional healing with a movement reeducation system. It is the least ideological healing system I have made contact with, and, like a living organism, integrates and evolves with the expansion of the healing field in general.

Proskauer: This type of massage, developed by Magda Proskauer, uses very light touch and derives its effectiveness from the relationship between breathing rhythm and the light touch of the technique. Clients claim that this experience is like an inner and outer massage.

Reichian Therapy: Developed by Wilhelm Reich (1898–1957), an Austrian psychoanalyst, this was probably the first Western body/ mind therapy to combine bodywork with Freudian psychoanalysis. Reich used manipulation to release blocked energy from structural disorders he called "body armor." During a Reichian session, the therapist may encourage intense movements to release pent-up anger and blocked energy. These movements may include stamping, kicking and tantrums. Many other bodywork systems, including Rolfing and Bioenergetic Therapy, and virtually all techniques that integrate body and mind, owe a debt to Reich.

Although the value of the Reichian system is now largely unquestioned, Reich's views originally were resisted by members of the medical establishment. However, many people who accept the concept of energy-based systems disagree with his underlying hypothesis that all blocked emotion is sexual in nature. Reich died in 1957 in a penitentiary, after his long-running conflicts with orthodox medicine led to his prosecution and conviction on charges of fraudulent medical practices. Reich's work and theories are generally held in high regard by most bodywork practitioners, and he is considered by many simply to have been a man ahead of his time.

Reiki: A light or non-contact approach to healing, actually a laying-on-of hands, based on ancient Tibetan and Japanese influences. Recent medical studies have shown it to be effective.

Rolfing: Originally known as structural integration, a system of deep muscular/connective tissue manipulation, it was developed by Ida P. Rolf (1896–1979). A researcher at Rockefeller Institute, she drew on her extensive knowledge of hatha Yoga to investigate the effect of structure on function. Rolf believed that, rather than coercing the body into submission, it should be encouraged to do what it really wants to do—work with, not against gravity. Moshe Feldenkrais has stated "when Ida Rolf integrates structure, as nobody else can, she improves functioning. . . . Rolfing was a revealing and unforgettable experience for me."

Shiatsu: Developed over the last three hundred years, this system, which means finger (shi) and pressure (atsu) is a Japanese-based bodywork system. The practitioner presses traditional acupressure points but may use fingers, thumbs and palms to diagnose and to free up energy blockages. Extensive attention is also focused on the interaction of expansive and contractive forces (yin and yang) that affect the flow of Chi (vital energy).

Swedish Massage: This is the system that most beginning students learn when they go to professional massage school. Its five basic movements work muscles to relax tension and promote blood and lymphatic circulation—a superb combination of relaxation and healing. It was created by Henri Peter Ling from techniques that he learned in China and then incorporated with Swedish gymnastic and exercise movements. Swedish massage consists of kneading (Petrissage), stroking (Effleurage), friction, tapping (Tapotement= percussion), and shaking or vibrating parts of the body.

Therapeutic Touch: This "laying-on-of hands" is based on the principle that health is promoted when there is a balance in the energy exchange between an individual and the surrounding environment. Therapeutic touch was systematized in 1971 by Delores Krieger, RN, Ph.D., who, after reviewing earlier research on healing, organized three pilot studies on the biochemical effect of therapeutic touch on humans. In this technique the practitioner passes his hands over the client's body and is able to sense energy imbalances which are expressed as electric shock, tingling, tightness, pulsation, heat, or coldness. Experiments have shown hemoglobin counts to rise dramatically after a Therapeutic Touch session. Because of Krieger's academic background and her teaching position in New

York University, Therapeutic Touch is now part of the curriculum at more than 30 nursing schools around the country.

Trager Psychophysical Integration: Developed by Milton Trager, a physician and former boxer, it involves a system of rocking motions, releases tension in the body and has an associated movement system called Mentastics. Once in Mexico I came down with a case of "turista" diarrhea from drinking the water. A Trager bodywork session had miraculous results.

Reflexology and Zone Therapy: These are two early American acupressure techniques that focus on points throughout the body but primarily on the feet. Reflexology focuses on the specific relationship between points found in the feet and various organs in the body. The basic concept of reflexology is that when a person applies pressure to the feet, he or she may notice a granular texture beneath the skin. Areas with extensive granulation are the most sensitive to the applied pressure. It is believed that this granular texture is a result of uric-acid crystallization in the feet. By rubbing out the crystals on the nerve endings in the soles, a reaction is initiated between these zones and associated organs and glands throughout the body. These reactions were called reflex reactions. Different theories abound as to why reflexology is so effective even if the uric acid theory does not hold up to present knowledge in anatomy and physiology. The point is that the system works well in relieving pain and many health problems.

HEALING TOUCH TECHNIQUES—YOUR FIRST EXERCISES

@ Energy Sourcing

Step 1
Sit comfortably on a chair, with both feet on the floor. Rest your elbows away from your body, not on your lap. Place your palms so they are facing each other. Now bring your hands close together as possible without touching. Separate them about two inches, then bring them together without touching again. Repeat this exercise. Can you feel heat, tingling or pressure between your palms or fingers?

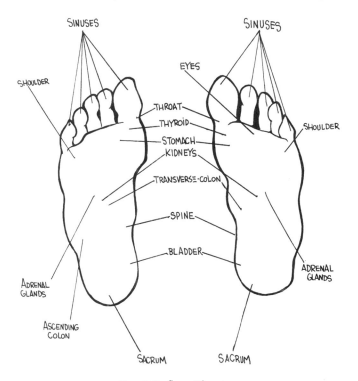

Foot Reflex Charts.

Step 2

Now place your hands eight inches apart. Slowly bring them toward each other at about two inches at a time. As they come closer, sense the field between them. Compress it as your hands move closer together. Focus your attention on this energy field. (A similar technique is predominant in the The Therapeutic Touch system developed by Dr. Delores Krieger.)

Step 3

Using your index finger, use firm pressure to locate the point of blockage. Ask your partner, "Is this tender to the touch?" or "Where do you feel pressure?" Direct your partner to let you know when you touch a spot that is more sensitive than the rest of the area. If you have enough sensitivity in your fingers, you will probably feel a thickening or tightness of the muscle. If you have difficulty locating the precise location with your index finger, use your thumb and then switch to your index finger once you have located the blockage.

Step 4

Now rest your finger gently on the point. Place your other hand on any joint of the body where it can rest comfortably. This second contact is made with the entire palm covering the joint and the fingers resting lightly on the body. Gentle pressure may be applied here but it is not necessary. This hand serves as an earthy, stabilizing factor to support and give structure and direction to the "Chi" as it flows through your body and emotions. Maintain touch until you sense warmth in your index finger—about two to three minutes.

Remember: This contact is a very subtle balancing tool. No benefit is gained from using pressure. Lightness of touch is the key.

@ *Light vs. Deep Bodywork*

Many bodywork systems lean toward an approach of gentle healing energy while others are a more invasive style of muscle manipulation. My own experience is that each has its place. Light work tends to have a more profound effect on emotional "holding patterns" and since light work is less invasive it enables the client to work through "emotional trauma" and structural blockages at an easier, more comfortable pace. Often emotional issues may be contributing to the structural situation.

There are, however, certain structural situations that seem to respond only to very deep and forceful bodywork. In these situations I may use a Shamanic Massage Technique called Connective Tissue De-armoring.

HANDS-ON HEALING AND SHAMAN MASSAGE TECHNIQUES

@ *Muscle Kneading*

The Muscle Kneading Technique should always be applied transversely (across the body of the muscle). If you place a lubricant on the skin you can press your fingers or knuckles parallel to the length of a structure (longitudinally). This follows the course of the blood and lymph vessels but does not greatly affect the tissue itself. This alternative to traditional Muscle Kneading is called Longitudinal Friction.

Though kneading increases circulation and is valuable to the deeper parts of the muscle, it also creates a difficulty since deep work and the resulting pain will cause the client to tighten up or contract the area being treated. This also reduces the benefits of the technique. The solution here is twofold. 1) The part to be worked on must be placed in a position that will leave it naturally limp. 2) The practitioner must integrate instructions to the client on visualization and diaphragmatic breathing to reduce the pain. (See the index for information on "Breathing" and "Visualization.")

Imagine yourself kneading bread dough and you have a sense of the finger and wrist movement that this technique requires. Used to stimulate the functions of the skin, Muscle Kneading is especially good for dry skin. In addition to the skin, it stimulates all vital functions of the body part where it is applied: glands, nerves, and blood vessels as well as muscles and connective tissue. It is the only technique in our system for which oil is used on the skin in order to reduce chafing and friction. After you apply a small film of aromatic oil to the skin, the kneading can begin.

Kneading is experienced by the body as an alternation between relaxation and compression. It helps to empty the blood and lymph vessels and to bring fresh fluids to these areas, thereby eliminating poisons and waste matter from the tissues and improving circulation. It is used routinely during warm-ups by dancers and athletes in order to reduce the possibility of injuries, cramps and muscle spasms.

Step 1
After applying a small film of aromatic oil on the area to be worked on, grasp the muscle with a squeezing action of your hand. If the muscle is properly oiled, it will immediately begin to slip out of your hand.

Step 2
As the muscle slips from your hand, quickly grasp it with your other hand. The muscle will continue to slide from hand to hand as it is pressed, creating a rolling effect. Continue the kneading for about thirty seconds to one minute for most areas, but for about five minutes on the back.

Step 3
Both you and the person you are working on should inhale deeply so that you may both take in the healing aromatic oils that will begin to fill the room from the friction of the kneading.

Muscle Kneading has many benefits. It is especially useful for firming weak muscles. Of all bodywork techniques, this is probably the most structurally oriented. It is invaluable in paralysis and in all cases where there has been tissue degeneration. It can be applied easily anywhere on the body with the exception of the shins, bony joints, and the skull.

In working with muscles near a bone that has been fractured, or near a sprain, Muscle Kneading is the technique to choose.

Caution: Avoid using this technique in any situation where deep pressure is ill advised such as hypertension, heart disease, cancer or irritated skin. Also avoid kneading on the fractured bone.

CHAPTER 3

@

TOOLS FOR HEALING HANDS

Healing Hands Through The Shaman's Tools

Shamanic tools serve as the keys that help open the doors to non-ordinary reality.

In order to give the best Shaman Massage session it is essential that you create an appropriate environment. This includes not only the necessary items such as oils, towels, and sheets, and equipment—a mat, massage table or on-site chair, etc.—but also of tools that will create a maximum quality experience for you and your partner. These include room temperature, lighting, aromatherapy, fresh flowers, colors, and choice of music.

@ Listening to Music

Listening to music is one of the most common forms of healing and relaxation. Each of us gives our own meaning to music. In the Shamanic tradition, music not only soothes through the outer ears but can be a vehicle for opening the inner ears as well. It is important, therefore, that you select music that you find peaceful and soothing but with which you also feel a deep intuitive connection. Certain musical pieces may carry a positive association with the past or have a spiritual sensibility. Certain notes, sounds and rhythms relate directly to the Chakras. In India people sing songs called Shabds that are said to have a power so uplifting that people slide out of their own bodies into a realm of wonder and mystic realization.

◉ Using Music as a Shamanic Tool

To use music to expand your healing potential, schedule a half hour of uninterrupted time. Don't answer the door; turn off the phone. Put on the music you have chosen, settle into a comfortable position, close your eyes, and take three long deep breaths into your abdomen. Mentally scan your body, noting areas of stress, pain and relaxation. Sense your emotional state and mood as you scan your body for tension. Listen to different parts of the music: the drumming, or rhythm or various instruments. Practice focusing from instrument to voice and onto other instruments. Each time a thought flows through your head, look at it in your mind's eye and then watch it float on as you bring your attention back to the music. Continue to breathe long, slow breaths. When the music ends, bring your mind back to your body, and sense how each part feels. What is your mood? Has it changed?

◉ Visualization

Visualization is a powerful tool for both client and practitioner in the structural and energy-based applications of touch.

In recent years the use of visualization and guided imagery as a healing and Shamanic tool has received a great deal of attention. Since the days of Mesmer (the French physician who rediscovered hypnosis), many physicians have known that very sickly and diseased individuals have gotten better and seen their health return as a result of hypnosis, visualization and other techniques based on the use of mental imagery. The power of visualization is not limited to health and healing. Many Shamanic practitioners use it as an essential element in the "vision quest."

◉ Why Does Visualization Work?

When you are involved in different mental activities your brain generates various types of wave patterns. These wave patterns have names such as alpha or theta. These different types of waves are produced in different areas of the brain at all times, but one or another type of wave tends to dominate when you are in each state of consciousness.

In a state of deep visualization, your brain generates alpha waves. These waves come at seven to fourteen cycles per second. The alpha waves of deep visualization are faster than the theta or delta waves of the sleep state, but are slower than the beta waves produced in the slow waking state. In recent years, clinical practitioners from many specialties and fields of thought have become interested in applying these tools to specific areas and situations including medicine, motivational training and psychology. Research has shown that functions that were generally believed to be involuntary, such as heartbeat and circulation, can now be placed to some level under our conscious control. Among the many areas where visualization and imagery have been successfully applied are in the treatment of stress and sleep disorders, sexual dysfunction and various medical problems including cardiovascular disease, hypertension, digestive disorders, cancer, diabetes, depression, medication dependence, phobias, and a variety of other disorders. It is no exaggeration to say that visualization and relaxation techniques may be among the most important therapeutic approaches that healers, physicians, motivational consultants and helping professionals of all philosophies and beliefs can offer the public.

@ How to Use Visualization Exercises

Visualization exercises can easily be done in just about any place and time and in only a few minutes. You begin by closing your eyes, getting into a relaxed position and starting to create mental pictures. Whether you apply the techniques in unison with a partner before the healing session, before going to bed, or when you wake up first thing in the morning, visualization is a powerful tool for connecting to your inner voice and for self-actualization.

@ Beginning Visualization Exercises

Visualization is most effective if done while you are sitting in a straight-backed chair, with both feet flat on the floor and your hands, palms up, and resting on your knees. Some people may find it more comfortable to begin with the palms resting down on the knees and this is certainly acceptable. If you are uncomfortable in a sitting position you may choose to begin visualization exercises while lying down. However, this is often not the most productive approach since you may fall asleep in this position. If you are in a place where sitting down is not convenient, visualization may even be done while standing.

As you begin to visualize you may find that your mind will sometimes wander. This is a natural occurrence and is nothing to become concerned or impatient about. If this does happen simply return to the image you had in your mind and continue a long slow breathing rhythm. You may even add to the environment by playing soft New Age music or Shamanic music.

@ Visualization Technique #1—Pain Control

Step #1—Find a quiet place where you will not be disturbed.

Step #2—Sit in a straight-backed chair, with both feet flat on the floor and your hands facing palms up and resting on your knees.

Step #3—Close your eyes and inhale and exhale long and slowly.

Step #4—As you are breathing deeply, slowly and rhythmically, visualize the area or part of your body where the pain seems to be centered.

Step #5—As you inhale, visualize that a blue light is entering your body by means of the breath and is surrounding and soothing the area of discomfort. Focus on this "blue energy" that is flowing into the pain and dissolving it.

Step #6—Now, as you exhale, clearly see in your mind that the feeling of pain is leaving your body as a gray cloud.

Step #7—Continue with this exercise until you feel relief and a sense of relaxation.

Step #8—Finish this visualization by taking a long deep breath, slowly exhaling and gradually opening your eyes. Remain quiet for a few minutes, becoming aware of your surroundings without getting up or moving around.

Step #9—Slowly begin to wiggle your toes and fingers.

Step #10—When you feel acclimated to the surrounding environment, you can arise.

@ Prayer

Prayer is an important element in healing and Shamanism. Prayer can be a call to the spirit world and to spirit guides and angels for help, verbal acknowledgment of one's relationship to the spirits, or a statement of appreciation for grace received.

Most people think of prayer as asking God for a favor. In the Shamanic approach the essence of prayer is that it is a means for connecting to your spirit guides and angels. The highest form of prayer is to surrender to the divine wisdom while asking for nothing in return. This surrender is the most sacred of relationships with your inner guides. It is what makes the prayer sacred or holy. For some Shamans, this surrender through prayer is the ultimate tool. For others it is in the repetition of divinely inspired words or sounds, given by initiation by a Shamanic elder or a living spirit guide (A sage in the Taoist sense, A Rebbe in the Jewish tradition or mystic master in the Indian tradition). This prayer of surrender is a sacred gift to the healing spirits in appreciation for their guidance or to request their guidance. But in the end even unanswered prayers are accepted as a Shamanic massage in themselves.

To pray is to be immersed in a sense of divine love. It is to tap into your inner truth, the truth that lies above the mental state. In true prayer you enter an altered state of consciousness. You forget your mind, your body and your own ego; in that you are connected to the divine consciousness, what Chinese Shamans call the eternal Tao.

The true prayer is one in which there is no false humility. You know that what you want may not be what you need and so you surrender the want. You give yourself completely unto the inner light. This is Shamanic actualization. In joyous and humble prayer you come in touch with healing "Chi." If you can have that feeling, then whatever you do guides you to the inner healer's voice, because you are a vehicle for the healing touch not the doer.

@ The Language of Color

Color is used in many ways in the Shaman's tool chest: through crystals, lighting of the bodywork environment, internal color images in creative visualizations, colored sheets and towels, and in the coloring imagery of music. The use of color in healing is directly tied into the five elements and healing through the Chakras. Reviews of classical and jazz concerts often describe the play of the instruments and the music itself in relationship to colors. Symbolism through language speaks of music as played in pastels, color-brilliant, light, dark jewel-like, and lustrous.

@ Lighting and Color

In some Shamanic processes, you will be using color visualizations and colored lighting. Specialized colored light bulbs are often valuable in removing the person from their normal environment and taking them to another emotional place.

If you are using standard lighting in the room, remember to

make it dim. Bright lights are glaring to the eyes and produce a sensation of harshness. You can completely dim the lights if you have indirect or natural light coming through a window. If you do all of your massage work in the same room, it may be valuable for you to use a dimmer switch so that you can adjust the intensity of the light.

@ The Bodywork Surface

One of the keys to healing with your hands is to create a healing environment. There are many effective tools for this purpose. Some of these tools have to do with the external environment and there is also the inner healing space. There are tools which will help you to come in contact with what many Shamans call "the light within us that heals." Through learning about and making use of these tools you will discover how your healing abilities can evolve through the simple act of touching.

The External Healing Space

There are three surfaces that you may choose from for Hands-On Healing. These are a professional therapist's table, a floor mat and a bodywork or massage chair.

@ The Healing Table

Professional healing tables are either stationary or portable. They should at a minimum be 6 feet in length and 28 inches wide. Portable tables are the most popular because they can be folded in half and transported and are easier to store than the stationary models. There are many additional features that can be purchased with a table. This of course increases the price, so for starters I recommend the most basic models. The essentials of any sturdy table should include cable supports on the legs for strength and stability, manual height adjustment, a face cradle, a washable vinyl covering, and thick padding for support and comfort.

@ On-Site Chairs

Some people are reluctant to get a massage because they are uncomfortable lying on a table or removing their clothing. Until the the mid 1970s, this posed an almost insurmountable problem for the massage therapist. However in the last few years various massage techniques have become popular that do not require the removal of clothing. Thanks to a massage therapist named David Palmer people no longer have to lie on a table to get massage and bodywork. David invented the original portable professional massage chair. This tool is a great alternative to the table massage. Some people need to sit upright, such as individuals with hypertension, certain circulatory, respiratory or heart conditions, people with limited mobility, and women in the last trimester of pregnancy. Chair healing is great for them. There are many different models of professional massage chairs.

If you are not prepared to purchase a professional chair but would like to work in a sitting position, you can use an armless straight-backed chair. Simply place some pillows on the front of the upright portion of the chair. Now have your partner face the back of the chair and lean against the pillows. In this position, you can comfortably massage his or her head, neck, shoulders and back as well as arms. Another approach is to place a pillow on a desk or table and have your partner sit on a stool and place their head on the pillow. There are also various types of foam head supports designed to be placed on desks or tables. These can usually be purchased from the same companies that sell massage chairs and tables.

@ Massage Mats

The simplest, easiest and least expensive way to practice Shaman is on a futon or exercise mat. Mats are light and thus easy to travel with. They require nothing more than a clean sheet and are easy to use for infants and young children. If you are working on an individual in a wheelchair or with a physical disability, a mat is the perfect choice.

@ Draping Material

A twin-size flat white cotton sheet or a large bath towel can be used to cover your partner during the session. White and 100% cotton is best because cotton blends and the dyes used to color the sheets may cause allergic reactions in some people.

◉ Room Temperature

Unless you are using a specific coolness or heat quality as part of the Shamanic experience, it is best to keep the room at about 70 degrees F.

◉ Massage Oil or Cream

Massage oils serve two fundamental purposes for the Shamanic practitioner: as a lubricant and for the inherent healing properties in the oil.

◉ Lubrication

Certain massage techniques require that the hands glide smoothly over the skin. Up until the 1970s most massage therapists used mineral oil as a liquid lubricant and corn starch or talc as a dry lubricant. As more massage therapists developed an interest in natural healing, talc and mineral oil (which is a petroleum by-product) fell out of favor and were replaced by plant-derived oils and lubricant creams. One of the benefits of plant-based oils is that they serve well as carriers for aromatic oils that may be used to create an altered state of consciousness. They can also be stored in a plastic squeeze bottle and are not as messy as creams. The bottle also keeps the oil free of contamination.

In recent years some massage therapists have begun to use what is called dry oil; a silicone-based, non-oily, quick-drying product. I have not been drawn to these since I find the plant-based "fixed oils" serve as the most effective carrying agent for aromatic oils which are valuable in Shaman massage. However, some clients react allergically to plant-based oils but are able to accept the dry oil lubricant.

Commercial massage creams or oils should be made from simple, natural, plant-derived ingredients. However this is not always the case. While exploring pharmacies and toiletry stores I have often found massage oils and creams that have a petroleum base, various artificial colors, preserving agents and other undesirable ingredients. Though naturally based oils can go rancid if not stored properly, a few drops of vitamin E in a newly purchased bottle of oil should extend its life. Many aromatic oils will keep rancidity from setting in as well.

@ *How to Choose a Lubricating Oil*

Even if an oil is natural it may not be appropriate for massage. Avocado and olive oils, for example, are too heavy in texture and pungent in aroma. Grape seed oil shouldn't be used on skin, since it can clog the pores and causes skin to break out.

Better choices are lighter oils, like sweet almond, hazelnut, and apricot kernel. There are a number of commercially prepared oils that contain concentrated extracts of flowers, plants, or herbs. These can be used, though you will find that when doing Shaman massage the most effective oils are those that are custom blended for each client.

THE FLOWER REMEDIES

@ *What Are They?*

Flower essences are vibrational-based remedies that seem to have a healing and balancing effect. They come in many forms—the 84 West Australian Flower Essences, the 5 Russian Flower Essences, California and Catskill Essences, and the group of remedies based on the discoveries of a young British scientist and homeopathic physician named Edward Bach. Over 50 years ago, Bach discovered that many of his patients' physical illnesses were directly related to emotional and psychological disturbances. Bach, a pathologist, immunologist, and bacteriologist, noted that resentment, anxiety, worrisome thoughts, even lack of self-confidence so depleted a patient's vitality that the body lost its natural resistance and became susceptible to a host of organic illnesses. Today research in the field of psychoneuroimmunology supports these findings.

Following extensive research, Bach found that certain species of wildflowers, when picked at a certain time in the blooming cycle and prepared homeopathically, possessed healing qualities. Bach eliminated those plants he found to be toxic or those which produce side effects, and ultimately succeeded in discovering 38 flowering plants, trees and special waters which were found to have a profound effect in stabilizing a wide range of mental and emotional stresses. Unlike chemical drugs which can be suppressive and create dependency, flower remedies, as they are commonly called, are considered completely safe, nonhabit-forming, and work by gently reestablishing emotional and psychological equilibrium.

The most famous of Dr. Bach's remedies is known in commercial form as Rescue Remedy or Calming Essence. This consists of five flower remedies (rock rose, clematis, impatiens, cherry plum, and star-of-Bethlehem) that Dr. Bach first used in the 1930s. It is especially effective in the aftermath of accidents and injuries, but also can counter the fear and anxiety of visiting the dentist or the mental stress and tension of dealing with bad news.

◉ Why the Flower Remedies Work

One theory is that flowers contain a subtle, vibrational energy that resonates with human emotions and feelings. Another theory is based on the belief that flower remedies can effect messenger molecules in the body's psychoneuroimmunity by altering key electrical impulses.

◉ How to Use the Remedies

The remedies can be purchased in most health food and natural food stores and pharmacies as tinctures and creams.

When you are ready to use the remedies, apply a few drops to your tongue, or put a few drops in a glass of water or tea and sip throughout the day. The remedies are extremely dilute and are harmless (though no more effective) in larger doses. Rescue Remedy and Calming Essence also come in a cream to be applied topically.

Considered a major breakthrough, these preparations are used by a broad spectrum of health care professionals worldwide, including Shamanic practitioners, massage therapists, healers, medical doctors, dentists, chiropractors, and psychologists, as well as the general public.

There is no single brand of flower remedy sold. They are prepared by different methods and different Shamans and healers around the world. Different manufacturers sell them under various names. What they all seem to have in common is that the remedies are a homeopathic-type solution prepared from the essences of certain flowers. In my own work I am most familiar with the flower remedies isolated and organized by Dr. Edward Bach. These are available from many health food stores and natural pharmacies throughout the country.

@ Opening the Shamanic Door

Any one of these flower remedies will begin the process of inner introspection:

Agrimony. For those not wishing to burden others with their troubles and who cover up their suffering behind a cheerful facade. They are distressed by argument or quarrel, and may seek escape from pain and worry through the use of drugs and alcohol.

Aspen. For those who experience vague fears and anxieties of unknown origin, and are often apprehensive.

Beech. For those who, while desiring perfection, easily find fault with people and things. Critical and at times intolerant, they may overreact to small annoyances or idiosyncrasies of others.

Centaury. For those who are overanxious to please, often weak-willed and easily exploited or dominated by others. As a result they may neglect their own particular interests.

Cerato. For those who lack confidence in their own judgments and decisions. They constantly seek the advice of others and may often be misguided.

Cherry plum. For fear of losing mental and physical control, of doing something desperate. May have impulses to do things thought or known to be wrong.

@ Stones and Crystals

Crystals are power spots, wherever they may be found. Shamans have been drawn to them due to their ability to concentrate and refract light. They are often used in energy focusing tools called pendulums as a source of energetic information. In this form crystals become power objects in the physical sense by opening the door to essential healing information.

Crystals and stones can be used in many ways to enhance healing. I use them by placing them directly on one of the five chakra points or by placing them on an energy center about an inch or two superior to the navel. Here is a description of some stones and their application:

Clear Quartz. Activates pineal & pituitary glands; stimulates the brain

Snowflake Obsidian. Benefits stomach & intestines; reduces stress

Rose Quartz. Helps kidneys & circulatory system; promotes fertility

Aventurine. Stimulates muscle tissue; eases anxiety

Tiger Eye. Strengthens spleen, pancreas, colon; grounds & centers

Rhodonite. Aids central nervous system, thyroid, pituitary

Amethyst. Strengthens endocrine & immune systems

Moonstone. Healing affinity with stomach, spleen, pancreas, lymph

Lapis. Strengthens skeletal system, activates thyroid

Black Onyx. Relieves stress; strengthens bone marrow

Leopardskin Jasper. Powerful healer; liver, gallbladder, bladder

Citrine. Good for kidneys, colon, liver, gallbladder, heart

Malachite. Strengthens heart, circulatory system

Red Jasper. Powerful healer; liver, gallbladder, bladder

Hematite. Activates spleen, positive effect upon bloodstream

Carnelian. Energizes blood; aids kidneys, lungs, liver

Sodalite. Aids pancreas, balances endocrine system

OTHER SHAMAN TOOLS FROM AROUND THE WORLD

@ *Medicine Bundle*

Some Native American Shamans carry this pouch or bag. Inside are sacred objects that contain or represent the spiritual powers he or she possesses.

@ *Power Objects*

These are sacred objects that a Shaman carries with him. These may be herbs, oils, prayer beads, crystals, prayers or any other number of sacred objects.

@ *Bull-Roarer*

A Bull-Roarer is a wooden Shamanic tool from the Aborigines of the Outback of Australia. When whirled in a circular motion, it makes an unusual primal sound vibration. It is believed that this whirling motion and the associated sound summons certain nature spirits.

@ Prayer Beads

Prayer beads are used throughout the world by medicine men and Shamans. Some beads are made of fine woods or precious stones, especially turquoise. In some cultures they were believed to have healing properties while in others possession of them could command honor or respect. The Mayans used turquoise as an offering to God, while some Tibetans strung 108 of them and used them to wear and chant upon. In many countries, turquoise is still used to protect humans and animals from harm. In North Africa, it was used to ward off the Evil Eye. In many cultures it is believed to preserve friendship and is a symbol of generosity and affection.

@ Sacred Images

In many Shamanic and spiritually based cultures, people may gaze upon a sacred image, icon or statue for various purposes. In Christian cultures many people will pray to statues of Jesus's mother, Mary. In many Asian cultures, especially Hindu and Buddhist traditions, staring at painted images is supposed to help one transcend all limitations. Paintings created for this purpose are called Mandalas. In Tibetan Buddhist traditions, Mandalas are meditated upon to raise one's consciousness. In the center of one such painting is the "Kalachakra," a sacred mansion and home of heightened consciousness and bliss. By visualizing and meditating on this mandala, it is believed that the seeds of enlightenment within your mind will be nurtured and will sprout and flourish. According to the Dalai Lama, the painting called the Kalachakra Thangka Print creates a favorable atmosphere that reduces tension and violence in the world.

Certain types of Mandalas contain geometric patterns. These are believed to assist the viewer in connecting to an inner Shamanic awareness. This ancient image is called a "Yantra." Looking directly at this combination of geometric patterns, subtle colors and spiritual imagery the viewer may experience a movement from mundane consciousness to an altered-consciousness experience.

◉ *Percussion Instruments*

Within many different Shamanic traditions the use of drums, rattles and other percussion instruments helps guide the Shaman student into an altered state of consciousness. If you wish, you can create your own from washboards, pots and pans, or any other objects. I listen to tapes of the African percussionist Baba Olatungi to get the feel of Shamanic drumming. His music is available in most record stores.

◉ *Rattle*

This is an instrument that is found in many indigenous cultures. It is shaken to produce clattering sounds. In specific Shamanic ceremonies the sound is believed to call the angels and spirit guides. The sound may help the Shaman to focus attention and shift into a non-ordinary consciousness especially for those about to go on a vision quest. Mexican Shamans are known to create a rattle out of a unique gourd that grows on a tree that grows high in the Sierra Madre mountains of southern Mexico. Though others have tried to locate this type of tree, only native Indians know where it grows. These rattles, used since pre-Hispanic days for healings, dance, ceremonies, and Shamanic rituals, are carved with various spirit animals and birds of the region. The gourds are sealed with a removable handle and the Shaman can add more sea shells, pebbles, or grains of sand to change or create a desired tone.

◉ *Breathing*

Once you have the external healing environment arranged, it is time to balance and open the internal healing environment. One of the key links between the mind and body, particularly between the emotions and the cardiovascular and sympathetic nervous systems, is the breath.

When we are experiencing fear, we hold our breath. When we have stress we may have a shallow breathing pattern. When we experience relief from a stress or trauma, we may take a deep breath.

In Western countries we don't usually equate breath and spirit, but in many other cultures the opposite is true. Sufis, a mystic Islamic group, base most of their spiritual practices on breathing.

◉ The Breath and Chi in Chinese Medicine

Breathing exercises form an important part of many Shamanic traditions. Indian yogis use breathing as an essential element to their internal balancing practices and in China the great book, *The Yellow Emperor's Classic of Internal Medicine,* indicates that therapeutic breathing and Tao-Yinn (Do-in) exercises existed seven hundred years before the introduction of Buddhism on the mainland of China.

The breath is one of the great Shamanic teachers. Each inhalation and exhalation produces amazing physiological responses. With each breath you inhale, your blood pressure rises slightly and arteries leading to the heart become narrower. Then you exhale, and with this action, your blood pressure goes down and your arteries dilate. As you retain each breath and retain the apposing emptiness each of these physiological states is maximized and then reversed. It is the ultimate expression of yin and yang, the opposing and at the same time merging forms of Chi, manifested in the physical form while residing in the spirit world.

To develop resistance against a disease, many healers in the Southern part of China love to balance and strengthen the internal parts of the body (nei-chung). This requires healing by breath as well as specialized exercises such as wringing out the hands and the crouching position (called seiza, etc.) to forcefully expel the disease.

In the 1970s I became familiar with the writings of the French obstetrician Ferdinand Lamaze. It was Lamaze who pioneered a technique in which a woman is trained to adapt her breathing to the various phases of labor. In this way the mother can reduce the pain of labor and facilitate a "natural" birthing process. In the Lamaze technique a woman in labor ceases fighting and resisting the birthing process. She surrenders to the body's natural functions. Reading Lamaze and tying his theories into my knowledge of pranayam (yogic breathing) and my own emotional experience, I was able to see the connection between a person's breathing patterns and emotional health. I began to recognize different patterns associated with breathing: yawning and sneezing repressed as social etiquette, and jaw muscles clenched to hold in powerful feelings. This connection of breath to emotion is so profound that when one is altered it immediately affects the other.

I also familiarized myself with the writings of Wilhelm Reich, the visionary psychiatrist and healer, and I explored his influence on the development of another system called Bioenergetics. Breath can stop emotion from being expressed; shallow breathing reduces awareness of feeling.

Effective breathing energizes and fortifies the body, balances the Chakras, opens the flow channels (meridians or nadis), clarifies our thinking, increases strength, stamina and endurance and promotes health and longevity. Sadly, few of us breathe properly. As with many biological processes, deep (diaphragmatic) breathing is something that children do automatically but that most adults have forgotten. "Taking a deep breath" may seem like the simplest thing in the world, but if you examine most people you would see that they take short breaths, breathing only from the chest or throat into the upper part of their lungs while the lower part of the lungs remain empty, essentially ignored. This shallow breathing is probably due to the tension and stress of our fast-paced life-style. The cost to our health is great. Shallow breathing does not bring enough oxygen into the body. Diaphragmatic breathing helps massage the internal organs and helps with the flow of blood and lymphatic fluids. Poor breathing patterns can lead to stagnation in the system and the buildup of toxic metabolic wastes that would be eliminated quickly through the internal massage motions that begin with the breath. Proper breathing will increase your focus and your reserve of life force and healing energy.

Shallow breathing patterns may also lead to poor self-image. Shallow breathers do not have much control over their voice. This may limit effective communication and create a poor image to others. They may respond with a body language that implies disinterest or disapproval, creating self-doubt in the speaker. Vocal control is important to communication, so much so that singing instructors train their students to breathe from the diaphragm. There are two elements to tapping into the healing breath: Depth and rhythm.

Elements of both the Taoist and Yogic traditions teach that the entire nervous system is nourished and balanced by a universal Chi found around us. In the early stages of creating a Shamanic sensibility it is valuable to reduce the rhythm of the breath from 15 to 20 breaths per minute to 5 or 6. After this is done, there should be a regulation of the rhythm of each respiration cycle so that inhalation and exhalation are equivalent in timing.

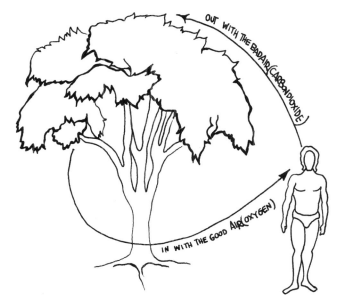

OUT WITH THE BAD AIR (CARBON DIOXIDE)

IN WITH THE GOOD AIR (OXYGEN)

Our Healing Breath Connects Us with Nature and Nature Spirits.

This process brings the body and mind to a state of complete resting. Indian Shamans and yogi's call this the "position of absolute rest," or Savasan. In this state there is a dramatic reduction of respiration rate, heart rate, and general body metabolism.

To begin this process place your hands on your lower abdomen and bring each breath to this area. As you do this you will automatically begin to shift into the proper rhythm. It won't happen instantly, but it will happen.

◉ Power Songs

The fullest expression of the breath as it links the ordinary and non-ordinary realities is through sound and song. As a child I would go to the synagogue on the Sabbath and watch the Cantor sing his power songs. The sacred words and tunes flowed through me and onward in waves of emotion.

I have listened to gospel and New Age music, and the drumming and singing of Baba Olatungi and his African drums. I have listened to "Amazing Grace," and the mystic poetry of the great Muslim sage-Shamans Kabir and Rumi. I have sat in intense meditation calling to the spirits all through the sounds of the power song. These power songs concentrate the Shaman's power and connection with the spirit guides. These are sounds of songs of humility and embracing of the inner divine. Find your own sacred songs. From your memories of church, temple or from the CD or cassette store, choose your sacred songs and sing them and play them before your healing touch sessions.

@ *Power Spot*

There are certain places where the universal Chi is richer, where the earth's healing energies are more accessible, more accommodating to the Shamanic seeker. These are the places where other worlds open, where non-ordinary reality opens the Taoist door to the source of healer's wisdom. The power spot is the place in nature where your angels and spirit guides dwell. It is a place where many Shamans retreat for ritual work. It is a place to withdraw the attention from the world and open the inner eye.

These are sacred sites. Not sacred in the sense that the physical ground there is holy but rather, like an acupuncture point on the body, these are the Chi centers of the planet. Jerusalem in Israel, Lourdes in France, Mt. Shasta, Mt. Rainier, The Dera in Beas India, The Black Hills and other mountain ranges, such as the Smokies, the Catskills, and the Santa Cruz Mountains, all in the United States, as well as the mountains of Tuscany in Italy. These have served as places of pilgrimage for Shamanic vision quests and spiritual retreats.

You do not have to visit these places to connect to your inner Chi. But they serve as symbol and metaphor for the holy place you can create in your own healing environment.

@ *Shamanic Dance and Movement*

Dance is used to honor the angels, devas, saints, personal spirit guides and the Shamanic process itself. Ecstatic dancing is a method used by Shamans in many cultures from Africa through Turkey to alter consciousness and merge with their helping spirits. During the dance the spirits move and dance through the body.

Dance calls on you to discover and explore your own Shamanic self. Gabrielle Roth, a great teacher and urban Shaman, sees the dance not just as physical movement but as an inner calling that you are responding to. She says, "It doesn't require going out and buying feathers or even beating a drum. But it demands listening to the beat of your own heart; finding your own rhythm; singing your own blues; writing your own story; acting out your own fantasies; and seeing your own visions. This is a contemporary, urban-primitive, Western-Zen, right-now trip. It's a journey into wholeness, an initiation into a Shamanic perspective."* You are, in a sense, dancing through this book as you flow rhythmically from chapter to chapter, technique to technique.

Exercise—whether it is jogging around the park, dancing to rock music or spinning flowingly to New Age sounds—is a powerful tool for opening the breath and freeing blocked "Chi." Balanced movement is a necessary part of the daily "rat race," and even at your place of work, a Tai Chi, dance or healing movement break is superior for increasing your physical, mental, and spiritual balance. It's definitely more balancing than a coffee break.

@ Homeopathy

Homeopathy is among the most respected and energy-balancing approaches available. Though its principles are thousands of years old and were used in ancient India and Greece, its present form was discovered and applied in the early 1800s under the name homeopathy from the Greek, *homoios* (similar) and *pathos* (suffering or sickness). Homeopathy is based on the law of similars, or as it was described in Latin "similia similibus curantur" (like things are cured by like). This concept of healing implies that a disease may be cured by a particular remedy if that remedy, given to a healthy person, produces symptoms similar to those of the disease.

When you visit a homeopathic practitioner, you will be asked to describe all of your symptoms and you will be asked many questions about your own and your family's medical history. Once the homeopath has the essential information, he or she will search for a remedy that has been shown under scientifically controlled conditions to produce a cure by matching your symptoms to the symptoms the remedy induces.

Generally speaking the best way to use Homeopathy for any chronic condition is by working with a practitioner who is skilled in choosing the appropriate remedies. For acute conditions, self-treatment is appropriate and there is no chance of using the wrong remedy and creating an unwanted side effect.

*Maps to Ecstasy: Teachings of an Urban Shaman, Gabrielle Roth with John London, New World Library, San Rafael, California, 1989, pp. 26–27.

@ Dr. Schuessler's Cellular (Tissue Salt) Therapy

The use of homeopathically prepared tissue salts was pioneered by Wilheim Heinrich Schuessler, a German medical doctor, physicist and physiological chemist. He developed this concept of healing in the early nineteenth century based on theories of his predecessor, Rudolph Virchow, a century before. Virchow discovered that the human body is made up of many tiny, living cells, which in turn are made up of water, organic substances, and inorganic substances. The inorganic substances, though present in very small quantities, were found to be essential to life. By Schuessler's time it was known that if the blood lacked one of the inorganic elements, the rebuilding and healing processes in the body could not take place. According to Schuessler, deficiencies in these vital substances eventually lead to a disease state. In Schuessler's time only twelve inorganic elements had been isolated in the cellular matter. Now many more of the elements are known, however most healers still use the Cell Salt Therapy with the original twelve tissue salts with which Schuessler worked. They are listed below:

Calcium Fluoride (Calc. Fluor.)
Calcium Phosphate (Calc. Phos.)
Calcium Sulphate (Calc. Sulph.)
Phosphate of Iron (Ferr. Phos.)
Potassium Chloride (Kali. Mur.)
Potassium Phosphate (Kali Phos.)
Potassium Sulphate (Kali Sulph.)
Magnesium Phosphate (Mag. Phos.)
Sodium Chloride (Nat. Mur.)
Sodium Phosphate (Nat. Phos.)
Sodium Sulphate (Nat. Sulph.)
Silicic Oxide (Silica)

There are many reference texts available in natural food stores describing which remedies work best with which conditions.

Both traditional Homeopathy and the Cell Salts system work extremely well with Hands-on Healing Techniques, especially Chi Balancing and Pressure Point Massage.

HEALING WITH CHI

When you can tap into Chi, you have connected to the ultimate healing tool. Chi is viewed differently in every culture, moves down different pathways, and is generally inaccessible in the traditional scientific view of what energy is. Whether seen as spirit, a reflection of spirit or something else, this "wireless anatomy" is common to all living things. In Chinese medicine, this energy circulates throughout the body along 12 specific pathways known as meridians.

These meridians are reflected on both sides of the body, flowing along the hands, arms, legs, trunk and head. In the Polarity energy-balancing system, they flow longitudinally, centrifugally, diagonally from joint to joint, and through energy centers down the center of the body called chakras. In the Chinese system, two pathways flow across the trunk, one in front and one in back.

In virtually all energy-based healing systems the wireless anatomy interconnects between all the different pathways. Some are primary and others are secondary. All interconnect, through the physical, emotional and spiritual realms. This interconnecting of energy and energy pathways creates a balancing of the expansive and

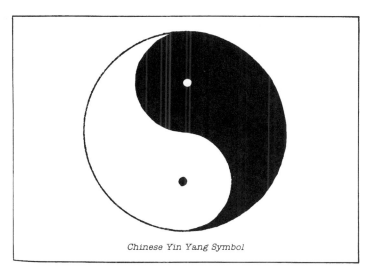

Chinese Yin Yang Symbol

Ordinary reality is a constant flow between expansive and contractive forces. This is well symbolized by the traditional Chinese Symbol for Yin/Yang.

contractive elements that are essential to all life. The circulation of Chi (Qi or Ki) is a response to the meeting point where centrifugal and centripetal merge; where hot becomes cold and vice versa; where expansive becomes contractive. This is called the balance of Yin and Yang.

When energy pathways are open, energy flows unobstructed and the life energy is balanced. The result is health and well-being.

To develop strength against an illness, the Southern Chinese focused on the internal parts of the body (nei-chung). Healing was accomplished by specific breathing (Ch'i meaning breath, air or life's energy) techniques twisting (wringing out) of the body and crouching position (seiza, etc.) for forceful expelling of the illness. This crouching position has much in common with the techniques used in Polarity Therapy. In this position there was a formation of three outer unions:

1. The shoulders united to the rib cage
2. The elbows united to the knees
3. The hands united to the feet

Within all Shamanic healing there is a process of balancing antagonistic-complementary forces. This frees up Chi. Chi stimulates the activity of all inner organs. When the circulation of Chi is blocked or there is a disturbance of its flow there is illness. In illness Chi may be depleted. We may regain Chi by absorbing external factors such as food, herbal medicine, aromatic oils, oxygen, light, sound, thoughts, vibrations, and transforming these into prana or Chi energy.

@ The Application of Chi in Daily Life

As you develop your inner-healing Chi you will begin to recognize that all healing comes out of a balance between the two cycles: **motion** and **rest.** By alternating between one and the other in a balanced rhythmic sequence, you can cleanse internal and energetic toxins from the Chi pathways and from the internal organs.

One way of balancing Chi is to sit in what Japanese healers call the seiza posture. In this position the junction of the toes is at the base of the spine. It is believed by many healers that this configuration enhances and recirculates the flow of Chi energy.

HANDS-ON HEALING AND SHAMAN MASSAGE TECHNIQUES

Massage and healing techniques that require finger pressure may include a wide ranging category of bodywork techniques and therapies that are used to stimulate or sedate the body's energetic flow. In addition to pinpointing energy blockages, Rhythmic Pressure Point Massage is also used to relieve deep-rooted muscle tension, structural problems and restrictions in the range of motion. Rhythmic Pressure Point Massage is the technique to choose for muscle spasms or cramps and is one of the main techniques for healing damaged tissue and reducing the formation of scar tissue after surgery or sprains.

During Rhythmic Pressure Point Massage, light, medium or deep pressure is applied with the thumbs, fingers, knees, elbows, or feet to key reflex points on the body. Some of these pressure points are the same as those used in acupuncture. Deep pressure tends to have a sedating effect while light pressure produces an energizing effect. The pressure effects life force in one's body by removing stagnation and energy blockages. This life force, or energy, encompasses all vital activities (spiritual, emotional, mental and physical).

There are various theories on why this technique is so effective. Some physiologists believe that pressure, even when light, somehow diffuses the lactic acid and carbon monoxide that builds up in muscle tissue. When these gases accumulate, they may contribute to stagnation of blood. When this happens a person may feel tired, stuffy and stiff.

@ Expanding the Internal Chi

1. Sit in the seiza posture.
2. Close your eyes and slowly scan your body from head to toe and back to head again.
3. Slowly and methodically focus on each muscle and sense how relaxed or tense it is.
4. As you find each tense muscle, inhale into it and allow it to relax.
5. Now repeat any of the following balancing words over and over as you observe your inhalation and exhalation. Composure (in Chinese, *shou*), Om, Name. Repeating any of these words at

each exhalation while sitting in the seiza posture will quiet the mind and relax the body.

⊚ Chi Balancing

Chi Balancing is best used with diaphragmatic breathing and visualization exercises.

Step 1
Sit comfortably on a chair, with both feet on the floor. Rest your elbows away from your body, not on your lap. Place your palms so they are facing each other. Now bring your hands close together as possible without touching. Separate them about two inches, then bring them together without touching again. Repeat this exercise. Can you feel heat, tingling or pressure between your palms or fingers?

Step 2
Now close your eyes and scan your body from head to toe. Focus on areas of stress, tension or pain.

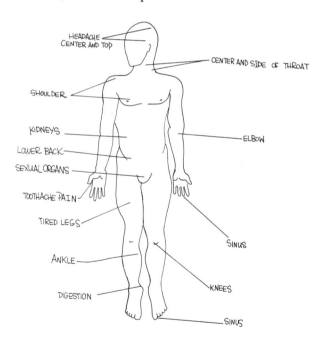

Reflexes: Sometimes pressing a point in one place affects a pain elsewhere in the body.

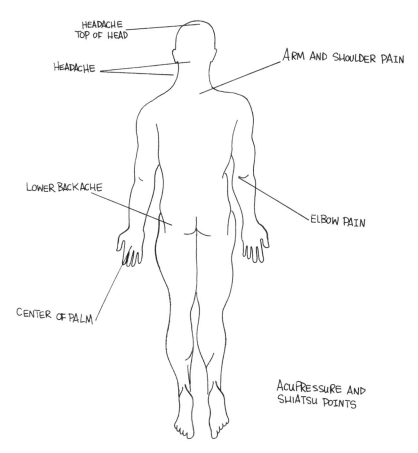

HEADACHE TOP OF HEAD

HEADACHE

ARM AND SHOULDER PAIN

LOWER BACKACHE

ELBOW PAIN

CENTER OF PALM

ACUPRESSURE AND SHIATSU POINTS

Reflexes: Sometimes pressing a point in one place affects a pain elsewhere in the body.

Step 3
Place your hands on the stressed area.

Step 4
Now breathe directly into your hand as it rests on the stress area and exhale out forcefully. Focus your attention on this process.

@ *Polarity Similars*

Polarity Similars is an extremely gentle technique. It is based on the concept that there is an energetic reflex action between certain body parts. By placing one hand on the point of blockage and the other on its corresponding reflex, the body's healing power is stimulated and the energy is balanced.

There are hundreds of Polarity reflex points. For simplicity and clarity, I am listing those reflex points that I have used most often over the years.

Superior Points (Toward the head)	Inferior Points (Away from head)
Fingers (each finger corresponds to a toe)	Toes
Palm	Bottom of foot
Forearm	Shin
Elbow	Knee
Upper arm	Thigh
Inside border of shoulder blade	Calves
Inside border of shoulder blade	Buttocks
Buttocks	Calves
Occipital bone	Sacrum
Sacrum	Back of heel
Shoulder joint	Hip joint
Wrist	Ankle
Mastoid part of temporal bone	Ischium
Parietal bones	Pubic bone
Jaw	Symphasis Pubis
Occiput	Sacrum
Sphenoid	Coccyx

Step 1
Find an area of discomfort and place your right hand over it.

Step 2
Place your left hand over the corresponding reflex points. Do this by laying your palms flat on your partner's body so that your entire hand is in contact with your partner's skin. Hold the contact for three to five minutes.

Step 3
A more specific, advanced and alternate technique is to heal using finger contacts. Make the superior contact, (the one close to the head) with the thumb or the index finger. The inferior contact, (the one farther from the head) should be made with the thumb or the middle finger.

Step 4
To increase the effect further, use Circular Pressure Point Massage described in Chapter 4 on these Polarity Similar reflexes.

Remember: When doing a Polarity Similars contact, it is important not to squeeze the body, and not to use heavy pressure.

◉ *Acupressure Massage*

The use of finger pressure instead of the needles used in acupuncture to effect energy pathways is a technique the Japanese have used for over 5,000 years. Shiatsu (finger pressure acupressure) is an acceptable medical practice in Japan and is authorized as a health treatment by the Japanese Ministry of Health and Welfare.

The acupressure that came to America after the Second World War was a different technique than traditional Japanese acupressure (Shiatsu). Western Acupressure is not one technique but rather includes Reflexology, Shiatsu, Polarity, Touch For Health, and various other systems.

Pressure Point Massage is a Shamanic approach to what is commonly called acupressure. This approach can be applied in a number of ways:

1. Jin Shin: A pattern of prolonged holding (one to five minutes) of key acupressure points along the meridians.

2. "First Aid": This approach is less concerned with balancing energy and focuses more as an instant approach to pain and discomfort. Specific points are pressed for the temporary relief of common problems such as backaches or menstrual cramps. I have developed a mapping of such points over the last twenty-five years.

3. Healing Through Movement. This is a means of balancing energy pathways through visualization, breathing exercises, stretches and postures. This is also known as Do-in.

◉ *Rhythmic Pressure Point Massage*

In addition to pinpointing energy blockages, Pressure Point Massage is used to relieve deep-rooted muscle tension, structural problems and restrictions in the range of motion. I usually define the amount of pressure I use by the terms "gentle," "firm," or "deep," but the amount of pressure will depend on your partner's

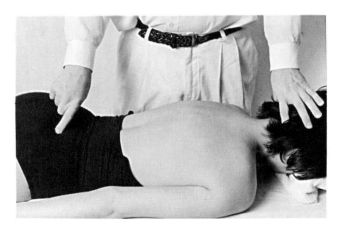

Polarity Similars: (Sacrum to occiput).

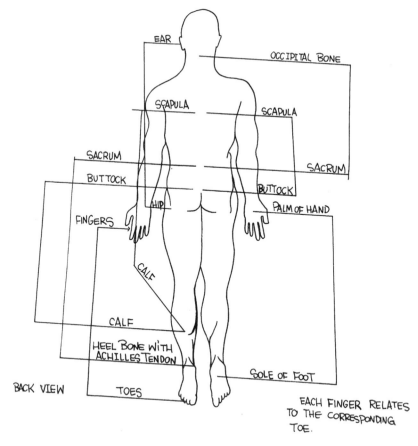

Polarity Similars, Back View.

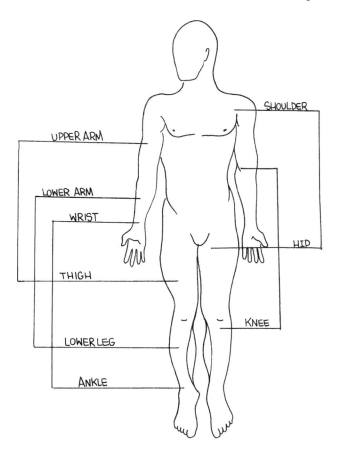

Polarity Similars, Front View.

tolerance for pain. Whichever pressure is used, the approach is the same.

Step 1
Use your thumb to locate the tightness or knot in the muscle. This spot will be particularly sensitive or will seem less pliant than the surrounding areas.

Step 2
Using your body weight, press your thumb into the area around the discomfort. Hold the pressure for a couple of seconds and release, then apply again. (In some situations, where you may wish

to exert less intense pressure, it is preferable to use the heel of the hand.)

Caution: Do not use this technique when the body temperature is higher or lower than normal. Never increase pressure suddenly—always apply it gradually, even when using deep pressure. And remember the guideline for applying pressure: never push forcefully with your finger. Instead, use your body weight to gradually increase the pressure.

CHAPTER 4

@

ANATOMY AND PHYSIOLOGY

To fully understand the therapeutic effects of Shamanic massage a familiarity with anatomy and how the body works is essential. Most of us fail to appreciate our bodies until something goes wrong.

Each action your body performs is a miraculous chain of reactions, whether what you are doing is simple or complex. From walking or sleeping to climbing or catching, each involves intricate messages and responses.

The body is comprised of several systems, which are made up of organs, which are formed from tissues, which are made up of cells. As you gain awareness of the body and its workings, you will develop confidence and control that will add a new dimension of satisfaction to your life.

THE ESSENTIAL ANATOMY

@ Cells

The physical basis of all life is the cell. It is the smallest living unit of the body. Cells perform a variety of tasks, and are different sizes and shapes. The largest cell in mammals is the ovum.

@ Tissues

Specialized tissues are formed by groups of similar cells. Each type performs a particular function. For our purposes the most important are:

- Bone tissue is hard connective tissue containing calcium and phosphate. Bone tissue loses these vital minerals as we age, and as a result becomes brittle and breaks easily.
- Epithelial tissue is a membrane that forms the covering over organs and body parts and provides insulation.
- Tendons and ligaments are soft connective tissue.
- Muscle tissue is made up of tough fibers which balance the structure of the body. It is the most abundant tissue we have. In most bodywork addressing poor muscle tone and fatigue and relieving tension are the primary concerns.
- Nerve fibers receive stimuli in the sense organs, transmit them from the sense organs to receptors in the brain, receive them in the brain and transmit them back again.

@ The Muscles

When we think about muscles we generally think about our outer musculature. These outer muscles include the hamstrings, the pectoralis major and the deltoids. What many of us do not realize is that deep in the center of the body there is another system of muscles. This system does not develop in a child unless that child begins to mirror people who exhibit and experience all aspects of body movement. If a child comes in contact with a piano player, a painter, a dancer or a crafts person he may begin to mimic the subtle movements in all of these actions. It is in this way that a child may integrate the knowledge of movement that brings deeper muscular activity into play. Some of these deeper muscles include the deep muscles of the back, the psoas, the muscles between the ribs (the intercostal muscles) and the pelvic rotators.

The outer muscles move at a faster rate than the inner ones and as such are suited for protection. When this protective quality expands beyond its effectiveness, it forms what many Shamanic practitioners refer to as body armor. Body armor can deaden your perception of the feelings of others and also limit your ability to express your own emotional feelings. Body armoring also restricts the proper functioning of the deeper muscles. The underdevelopment of deeper muscles can reduce the quality of our physical health and our emotional clarity.

The primary structural factors that define the state, position and functioning of the various body systems include fascia, muscles, tendons, ligaments, cartilage, and bones. With the exception of muscle tissue, all tissues consist of the same primary material: reticular fibers, collagen, elastic fibers, and a gelatinous medium. Ligaments are different from tendons because the amount and proportion of these components differ and this applies to all other tissues as well.

@ *Body Structure and Fascia*

The myofascial system—the combination of fascia and muscle—is an essential element of the body's structural foundation. It not only supports and protects the vital organs and glands, but its integrity defines and determines how the muscles in the body function and how all systems that are based on muscular function are interconnected. The body is not a collection of parts that work together as in a car engine. Rather it is an integrated physiologic system where a shift in any of its elements will affect all the others. On a structural level this interaction includes the nervous system and the quality of movement in the joints. Emotional or physical stress can leave its imprint in the fascia and create pathways that over time will create resistance and limitation of both physical and emotional flexibility.

The myofascial system and its related neural mechanisms determine spatial movements of joints and thus the direction and quality of all movement. In turn, movement acts as a pumping mechanism; in this way, the myofascial system is an important factor in fluid exchange at all levels of the organism. Anatomically, the myofascial system thus has a part in determining metabolic levels in local areas as well as in the body as a whole. It also becomes a vital factor in the bioenergetic regulation of the body and its thermodynamic and homeostatic equilibrium.

We tend to think of bones as the hard, white, bleached forms we saw hanging in our high school and college classrooms. Unfortunately we cannot easily see living bone. If we could, we would see resilient forms covered with vascular membranes, the periosteum, with many blood vessels at their ends; capable of healing the most serious fractures.

@ *Organs*

While cells form tissues, tissues form organs. Unlike the similar cells which make up tissues, organs are composed of several differ-

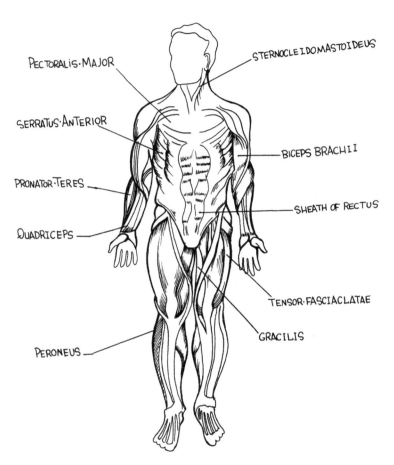

PECTORALIS·MAJOR

STERNOCLEIDOMASTOIDEUS

SERRATUS·ANTERIOR

BICEPS BRACHII

PRONATOR·TERES

SHEATH OF RECTUS

QUADRICEPS

TENSOR·FASCIACLATAE

GRACILIS

PERONEUS

The Muscular System, Front View.

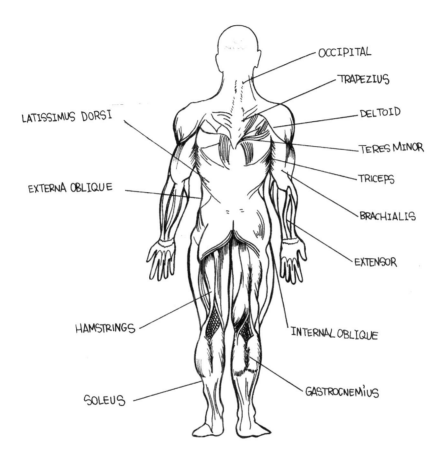

The Muscular System, Back View.

ent kinds of tissue. The main organs are the skin, heart, kidneys, lungs, stomach, liver, gallbladder, spleen, and pancreas.

The skin is the largest, heaviest organ of the body. On an average adult male it measures about seventeen square feet. There are millions of cells forming various tissues, several feet of nerve fibers and minute blood vessels, one hundred sweat and oil glands in one square inch of skin.

Skin protects the body against parasitic invasions and injuries, aids in elimination of wastes, regulates body temperature, stores food and water, prevents too much loss of fluid from the body, receives sensations, and conducts vitamin D when exposed to the sun.

Skin has an outer layer, the epidermis, and an inner layer, the dermis, which lies beneath. The epidermis is made up of layers of cells from which dead cells are continually shed. The dermis contains nerve endings, hair follicles, capillaries, sweat glands, and sebaceous glands, which secrete through the epidermis to maintain its elasticity.

There are numerous disorders of the skin. They include: blackheads, acne, hives, eczema, and rashes from allergies or infectious diseases, as well as moles, small blood tumors, cancer, warts, boils, and ringworm.

There are many Shamanic massage techniques described in this book which may be used without complications when skin disorders are present. Note that traditional Swedish massage involves quite a bit of rubbing and kneading of the skin and is not recommended for most skin disorders.

SYSTEMS

Organs work together to form systems, the human organism is a complex collection of these systems. Some are visible and some are invisible. Each system performs a specialized task. The digestive system for example, includes the mouth, salivary glands, pharynx, esophagus, stomach, large and small intestines, pancreas, liver, gallbladder, and appendix.

Some systems are more readily affected by Shamanic massage than others: skeletal, muscular, circulatory, nervous, respiratory, digestive, and urinary.

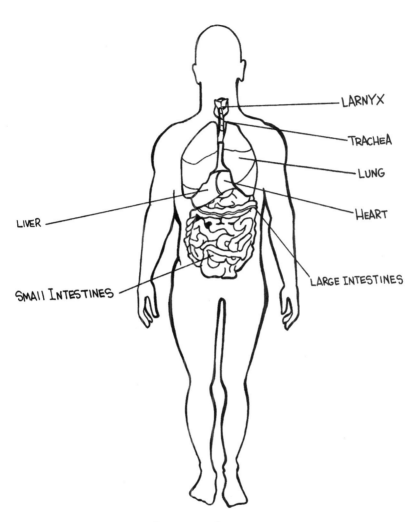

The Internal Organs.

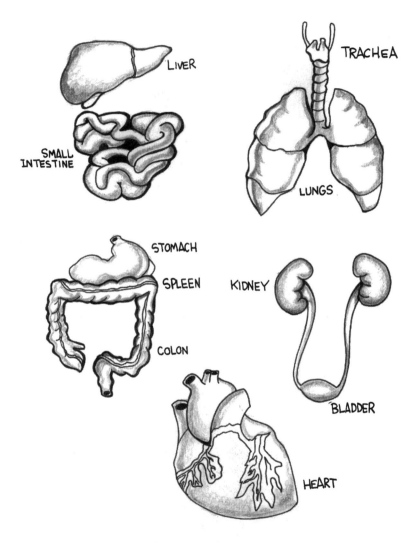

The Internal Organs.

@ The Skeletal System

The skeletal system is comprised primarily of bones and cartilage. It supports the body, as a frame supports a house. It works together with the muscular system to provide movement and flexibility. It also protects the soft, easily damaged internal organs.

Bones are classified as either long, short, flat, or irregular. Generally long and short bones are associated with movement, while irregular and flat bones protect the internal organs. For example, the femur and humerus, which are located in the leg and the arm, are long bones, and allow the limbs to move as they do. But the bones of the skull are flat, and protect the brain. Shamanic massage affects bones by aligning the muscles and tissues around them to provide better support for movement and balance.

It is a joy to view the flexibility of the human body when you realize how intricate the network is between bones, muscles, ligaments and tendons.

- Each foot has thirty-two joints and twenty-eight bones.
- Each hand has twenty-seven bones and thirty-two joints.
- The spinal column has 134 movable joints, not counting the intervertebral disks.
- The pelvis consists of three joints: two sacroiliac joints and one right in the middle of the pubic bone.
- Sixteen bones in the skull, and nearly fifty joints.

At one time it was believed that the pelvic bones were immovable. However in recent years it has been found that individuals who have a well balanced pattern of breathing, body movement and receive appropriate manipulation (bodywork) have mobile pelvic joints.

@ Cartilage

Cartilage is soft connective tissue. It covers the joints between the bones and is easily damaged. It is affected by impact and improper movements which can tear it, and diseases of the joints such as osteoarthritis. Shamanic massage and exercising in water can help to tonify and strengthen cartilage.

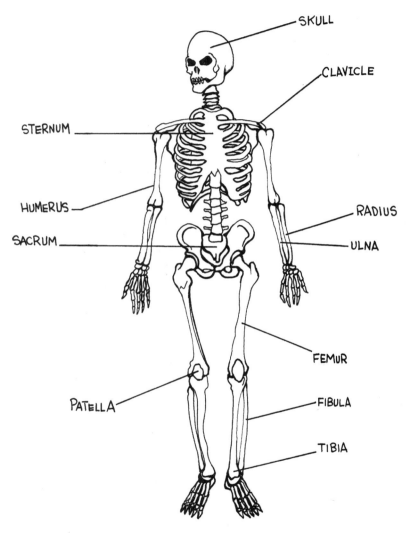

Skeletal System, Front View.

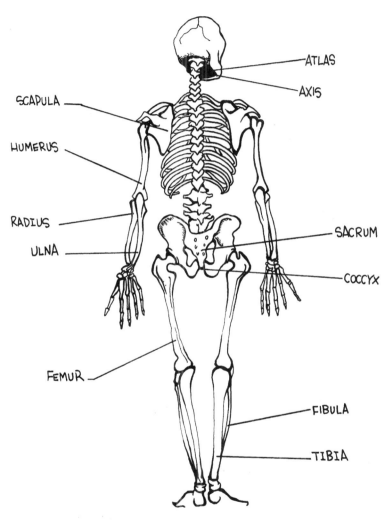

Skeletal System, Back View.

◎ Joints

Joints are the points of connection between the bones. They are classified as immovable or freely movable. Flexibility and strength of the joints are determined by the surrounding muscles, tendons, and ligaments. Tendons attach bones to muscles, ligaments attach bones to other bones. Many joints have extremely limited movement, such as the sacroiliac, in the pelvic girdle between the sacrum and the ilium. The only time this joint moves is during birth. A hormone is released during pregnancy which relaxes the strong ligaments that hold the sacroiliac in place. This allows a spreading of the bones and the joint's movement for delivery. The freely movable joints are more important to body movement and Shamanic massage.

MAJOR SKELETAL BONES

◎ Skull

This bony framework of the head consists of eight flat cranial bones that protect the brain, and fourteen facial bones that create the contours of the face. In some bodywork systems there are specific cranial manipulations. Many practitioners believe that lower back pain, specific vision problems, neurological imbalances, sacral problems, and foot and respiratory imbalances are directly affected by adjustments to the cranial and facial bones.

◎ Spinal Column (Backbone)

This central structure of the skeletal system is the major support for the head and trunk. It protects the delicate and highly sensitive spinal cord. The spinal cord carries nerve impulses to and from the brain. It also controls the activities of organs, glands, and muscles. Spinal cord damage often results in partial or total paralysis.

The spinal column consists of 26 movable vertebrae: 5 in the lower back (lumbar vertebrae), 12 in the upper back and chest (thoracic vertebrae), and 7 in the neck (cervical vertebrae), and 2 other movable vertebrae at the base of the spine, (sacrum and coccyx).

The first cervical vertebra is known as the atlas. It connects with the occipital bone of the skull, which forms the back of the head. The second cervical vertebra is the axis. The others are designated by number from the occipital bone down (e.g., third cervical vertebra, fourth cervical vertebra, etc.).

The 12 thoracic vertebrae are attached to the 12 pairs of ribs. The vertebrae support the upper back and chest, and the ribs protect the lungs.

The lower back is made up of the 5 highly mobile lumbar vertebrae. Before being passed down to the feet, over half of the total body weight is carried by these vertebrae. The powerful lower-back muscles, abdominal muscles, buttocks, and legs support the lower-back area. This area is vulnerable to physical stress from bending, bad posture and poor walking and sitting habits. Lifting too much weight can cause ruptures and hernias, impact can cause rotation and slipping.

The sacrum is located between the fifth, or lowest, lumbar vertebra and the coccyx. Its triangular shape makes it look like one bone, but it is actually five fused vertebrae. Many of the effects of bad posture show up here, because body weight is distributed to the hip joints via the sacrum's connection with the pelvic girdle.

The coccyx (tailbone) is a another small, triangular bone attached to the bottom of the sacrum. It consists of four tiny, fused vertebrae. Most allopathic health professionals think it is functionally unimportant, but the sacrum, coccyx, and pelvis are major storage areas for vital life energy. When body manipulation techniques are applied to these areas, rapid energy balancing as well as structural changes may be brought about.

The entire spine is a major holding place for tension. The chiropractic, osteopathic, and Naprapathic systems believe health problems are caused by imbalances in the spinal column. In Shamanic massage we acknowledge the importance of the spinal column, but have a different approach. For example, in chiropractic philosophy correcting the position of the vertebrae is believed to affect nerve and muscular functioning, whereas in Shamanic massage we believe stabilizing the muscles causes the vertebrae to correct themselves. Some exercises have similar effects. Though chiropractic and osteopathic manipulations work very well for back problems and migraine headaches, many practitioners have begun using complementary techniques, particularly kinesiology, for other problems.

◉ *The Clavicle*

The clavicle (collarbone) is a straight bone joined to the scapula (shoulder blade) at its outer end and to the sternum (breastbone) at its inner end. Special care should be taken when doing any bodywork around the clavicle because it is fragile and cannot endure heavy pressure.

◉ *Ribs*

The ribs protect the lungs, heart and other essential areas in the chest. Of the 24 ribs, the first 7 pairs are connected to the sternum (breastbone) with cartilage. Pairs 8 through 10 are connected to one another by a continuous cartilage rather than to the breastbone. Rib pairs 11 and 12 (floating ribs) attach only to the thoracic vertebrae. If the ribs are moved, or cartilage tears or is damaged, massage and body manipulation is often valuable.

◉ *Diaphragm*

Although the diaphragm is the most important muscle involved in breathing, the muscles of the chest cavity, between the ribs (the thoracic wall), also play an essential role.

◉ *Sternum*

The sternum (breastbone) is a flat bone at the front of the chest area which stabilizes the ribs. Fractures of this bone generally heal without trouble, but the heart lies directly behind it, so it is wise to use caution when doing massage and bodywork in this area.

◉ *Scapulae*

The scapulae (shoulder blades) are a triangular-shaped pair of bones in the upper back, on either side of the thoracic vertebrae. They are each about the size of a hand. While most of the bone is very thin, the outer border is rounded and stronger, and embedded in powerful muscles.The scapulae are well padded, and not often broken.

If the muscles along the insides of the scapulae are tight, this generally indicates imbalance in the respiratory or digestive system.

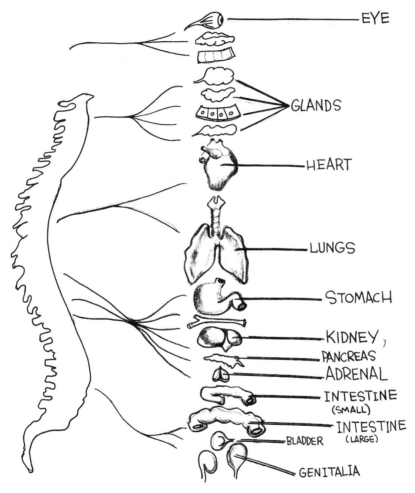

— EYE

GLANDS

— HEART

— LUNGS

— STOMACH

— KIDNEY,

PANCREAS

ADRENAL

INTESTINE
(SMALL)

INTESTINE
(LARGE)

BLADDER

GENITALIA

Pressure on Spinal nerves by the Vertabrae may have a negative effect
on organs and glands.

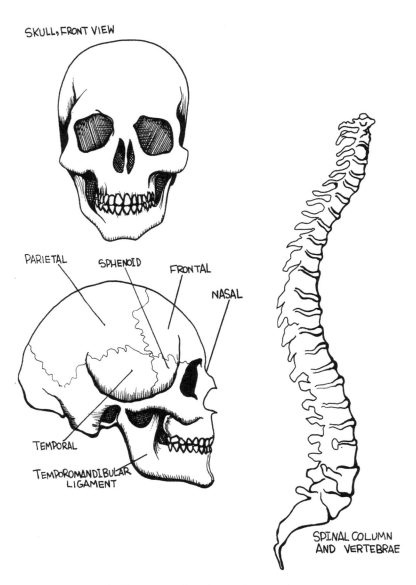

SKULL, FRONT VIEW

PARIETAL   SPHENOID   FRONTAL   NASAL

TEMPORAL

TEMPOROMANDIBULAR
LIGAMENT

SPINAL COLUMN
AND VERTEBRAE

Skull, & Spinal Column & Vertabrae.

Relaxing these muscles through Shamanic massage techniques will relieve many problems associated with digestion and respiration.

@ *The Pelvis*

The pelvis is actually a large pair of bones, located near the center of the body. The pelvis attaches the spine, sacrum, and femur (upper leg bone). The weight of the upper body balances and pivots around on it. Pelvic injuries can leave you temporarily immobilized, but they can often be helped by body manipulation and rest.

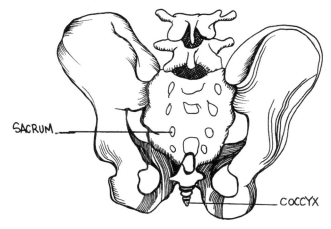

Sacrum and Coccyx.

THE ARMS AND HANDS

The Humerus is a major skeletal bone in the upper arm. It fits into a shallow socket in the scapula at the shoulder, forming the shoulder joint. It is easily dislocated from the shoulder socket. Breaks are common and heal when the bone is set. Bear in mind, when massaging the areas around a newly healed bone, that the muscles may be weak from lack of use.

The Ulna and Radius are the two bones of the forearm. The ulna forms the bony projection at the elbow and is the longer and thinner of the two. Strain falls on the radius at the wrist. If one of them is broken, the other is usually affected.

The Carpals are the eight bones that form the wrist. They are connected to the metacarpals, which are then connected to the phalanges. Surrounding muscles and tissue benefit from Shamanic massage because it can alleviate pain and stiffness at the joints.

The Metacarpals are the five bones which lie between the wrist and fingers.

The Phalanges are the fourteen bones on each hand that form the fingers, and the toes on each foot.

THE LEGS AND FEET

The Femur is the longest bone in the body. It connects the hip joint and the knee joint. The top of the femur breaks easily when impacted. It is especially vulnerable in elderly people. Increased

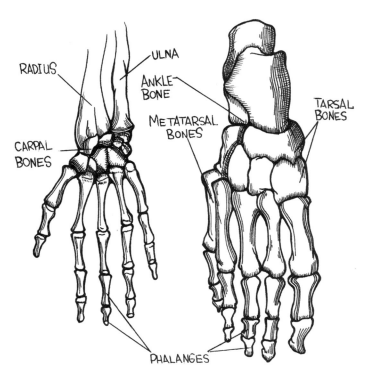

Bones in Wrist and Hand/Bones in Ankle and Feet.

fragility of the bones in older people is usually made worse by bad dietary habits.

Note: Osteoporosis weakens the bones. The use of cortisone for the symptoms of osteoarthritis and other health problems can often aggravate them or even cause long-term side effects.

The Fibula and Tibia are the two bones between the knee and ankle. The tibia, or shinbone, is the larger one. The smaller fibula anchors the upper leg to the ankle. It is easily broken.

The Tarsals are the seven bones of the ankle. The muscles around the ankle can become stiff. Blockages may impede blood flow, as in the carpals or wrists. Pain or discomfort results, but is helped by Shamanic massage techniques.

The Metatarsals are five bones that form the metatarsal arch and the ball of the foot.

@ The Muscular Physiology

Muscles comprise at least two-fifths of the total body weight and are the most abundant tissues in the body. They contain nerves and blood vessels. They facilitate body movement because of the following characteristics:

- **Contractility:** the capacity to shrink or contract inherent in all cells. Muscle cells are specialized to contract in length, but not width.
- **Extensibility:** the capacity to stretch. Stretching movements are important for muscular health because when a muscle is stretched it contracts easily and with greater strength.
- **Irritability:** the capacity to respond to stimuli. The muscles contract when chemicals, heat, electrical shock, or pressure are applied.
- **Elasticity:** the capacity to convey an impulse. When muscle contracts, the fibers tense and pull the bones together. This results in movement.

Note: Flaccid or fatigued muscles may have difficulty contracting. Flaccidity is caused by non-use. Excessive use depletes the muscles of oxygen and builds up lactic acid (a waste product), causing fatigue.

@ Remember: When Giving Shamanic Massage:

- Muscles usually act in groups.
- Muscles move the bones or body parts located directly above or below them, e.g. neck muscles move the head; thigh muscles move the lower leg.
- Muscles' expansive and contractive properties produce heat. They determine the body's form and posture. A person with good posture often seems more dynamic, regardless of other physical characteristics, whereas a physically beautiful person with poor posture can seem less attractive.
- Many muscles need attention because of stored stress, flaccidity, or fatigue. Manipulation or Shamanic massage helps maintain flexibility, vitality, and balance.

@ Here is a list of terms describing muscles based on the type of movement they produce:

Supinator:	Turns the palm of the hand upward.
Pronator:	Turns the palm of the hand downward.
Flexor:	Bends a body part.
Extensor:	Extends a body part.
Adductor:	Draws a body part toward the midline.
Abductor:	Draws a body part away from the midline.
Levator:	Raises a body part.
Depressor:	Lowers a body part.
Sphincter:	Opens, closes or reduces the size of an opening.
Tensor:	Makes a body part tense or rigid.
Rotator:	Rotates a body part on its axis.

@ The terms below describe various positions of the body. They are useful when locating specific parts or imbalances:

Exterior:	The surface of the body.
Interior:	Inside the body.
Anatomic Position:	Facing the observer with palms turned forward.

Superior:	Toward the head.
Inferior:	Toward the feet.
Anterior:	Toward the front of the body.
Posterior:	Toward the back of the body.
Medial:	From head to foot, down the center of the body.
Lateral:	From the midline to the outside, across the body.
Median:	From the outside to the midline, across the body.
Proximal:	Closer to the point of attachment.
Distal:	Farther from the point of attachment.

THE CIRCULATORY SYSTEM

The circulatory system transports blood and lymph throughout the body. Blood carries oxygen and nutrients to the body cells, removes wastes, aids in the regulation of body heat, and energizes the body. Lymph cleanses the system and protects the body from disease.

From the heart a web of arteries and capillaries feeds blood to all the parts of the body, veins carry it back. The heart forces oxygenated blood out of the left ventricle, through the aortic valves and into the aorta, from which the arteries branch out into the body. The smallest branches of the arteries are tiny blood vessels called capillaries, which in turn lead to veins. Veins merge to form the inferior vena cava and superior vena cava, which return deoxygenated blood to the right auricle of the heart from the trunk, legs, head, neck, and arms.

Contraction of the right ventricle forces blood through the pulmonary valves into the pulmonary arteries, which carry blood to and from the lungs. The lungs remove carbon dioxide from the blood and replace it with oxygen. Oxygenated blood then returns through the pulmonary veins to the left auricle of the heart, then passes through the bicuspid valve into the left ventricle, which again sends it into the aorta, where the process starts over.

◉ *Lymph*

Lymph is a slightly yellow fluid. It aids in the production of white blood cells, which combat infections. Blood plasma filters through the capillary walls into spaces between the cells and becomes lymph. Drained by lymph capillaries, it circulates via a network of small vessels or channels.

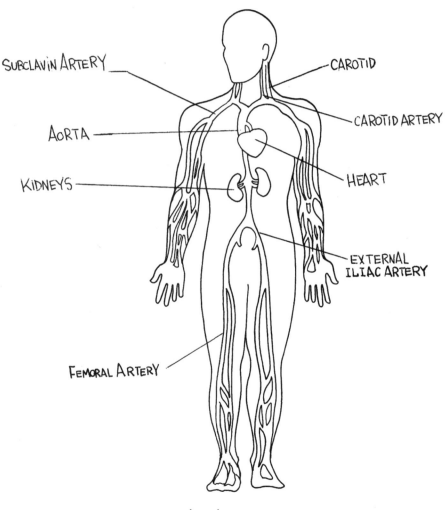

Arteries.

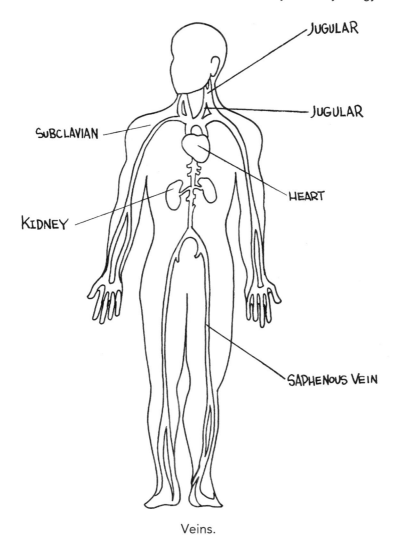

JUGULAR

JUGULAR

SUBCLAVIAN

HEART

KIDNEY

SAPHENOUS VEIN

Veins.

Lymphatic tissue, called lymph nodes, are found in groups at the armpit, neck, groin, abdomen, and chest area. Lymph nodes filter waste particles and bacteria to prevent them from entering the bloodstream. They can become inflamed and swollen and are then easily felt through the skin.

Structural causes of inflammation, such as carrying a heavy bag only on one shoulder, can imbalance the lymph nodes under the arm. It is possible to increase the swelling with massage, so check to see if the cause might be structural. If not, Shamanic massage can help the blocked gland to open, and allow the lymph to flow freely again.

Lymph drainage depends on the contraction of muscles. Immobility due to pain or paralysis seriously interferes with proper drainage.

@ Shamanic Massage Benefits the Circulatory System by:

- Assisting movement of lymph through kneading on the inside of the thighs from the knee up to the pelvis and under the armpits. This has a strengthening effect on the immune system and improves the elimination of waste.
- Easing stress on the heart by pushing the return of blood to it. Very helpful in cases of forced inactivity due to illness or injury.
- Improving blood circulation and relieving venous and lymphatic congestion.
- Increasing supply of oxygen and nutrients to all the body's cells.

THE NERVOUS SYSTEM

The nervous system regulates and coordinates other systems and organs. It comprises the central nervous system, including the brain and spinal cord, and the autonomic nervous system, consisting of groups of nerve cells and nerves.

Nerve cells, or neurons, conduct electrochemical energy called nerve impulses. When a smell or color or tickle is perceived, it is the result of sensory nerves transmitting impulses to the brain from the sense organs: the skin, eyes, ear, nose, and taste buds. To move the body or respond to a stimulus, motor nerves must carry messages from the brain to the muscles.

The central nervous system coordinates energy, movement and thought. The nervous system stimulates and triggers the emotions. Its messages guide the body and mind. Faulty connections between mind and body can cause conditions like cerebral palsy, in which the mind functions fully, but cannot control the body. In cases where the reverse occurs, the mind does not function and can't send signals to the body. The muscles may be spasmic and uncontrolled. Shamanic massage can relax the muscles and help train them to be controlled.

Note: Shamanic massage can be used to relax the nerves and ease stress. In cases where there is sluggishness and mental drowsiness, a tonifying massage can perk up the entire system.

IMPORTANT PARTS OF THE NERVOUS SYSTEM:

◉ *Cerebrum:*

The cerebrum controls conscious, voluntary processes. It is the largest structure of the brain.

◉ *Cerebellum:*

The cerebellum is the section of the brain behind and below the cerebrum. It is responsible for the coordination of complex muscular movements such as playing an instrument, dancing, and sports.

◉ *Cerebral Cortex:*

The cerebral cortex is the gray tissue forming the outer layer of the cerebrum. It's responsible for some higher functions: talking, thinking, memory, and judgment.

◉ *Thalamus:*

The thalamus is a large, gray mass of tissue located at the base of the brain. It sends sensory stimuli to the cerebral cortex for interpretation. The thalamus also appears to be involved in emotional responses and the integration of speech.

◉ *Hypothalamus:*

The hypothalamus lies below the thalamus. It regulates body temperature, water balance, sugar and fat metabolism, and endocrine gland secretions.

🌀 Spinal Cord:

The spinal cord is a column of nerve tissue from the brain to the second lumbar vertebra. All nerves to the trunk and limbs originate at the spinal cord, the center for reflex actions.

🌀 The Autonomic Nervous System:

Controls the unconscious and involuntary body functions: the glands, the heart muscle, and smooth muscle tissue found in the walls of the digestive organs and blood vessels. There are two sections: the sympathetic and the parasympathetic.

🌀 The Sympathetic Nervous System:

Controls stress reactions. It initiates the "fight or flight" response during which the release of adrenaline prepares the body for action by causing increased heart and respiratory rates, sweating, dilation of the pupils, and increased flow of blood to the skeletal muscles.

🌀 Parasympathetic System:

This system controls normal body functions such as digestion, absorption of nutrients, draining of the bladder, and the reduction of heart and respiration rates.

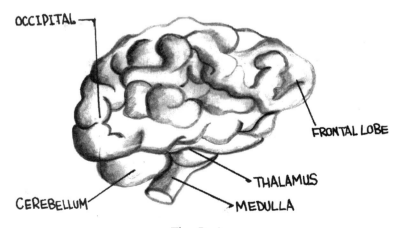

The Brain.

@ *Shamanic Massage Benefits the Nervous System by:*

- Sedating or stimulating the nervous system, depending on what is needed and the technique used.
- Balancing the nervous system, affecting all the systems of the body.

RESPIRATORY SYSTEM

The respiratory system consists of the nasal passages (nose), pharynx (throat), larynx (voice box), trachea (windpipe), bronchi, lungs, and diaphragm.

By respiration, air enters and exits the body. In the lungs oxygen is absorbed by the blood, which then distributes it throughout the body. The blood picks up carbon dioxide and takes it back to the lungs to be exhaled along with water. Each breath brings a fresh supply of air to the lungs, but some air always remains in them.

The muscles involved in breathing are those of the chest cavity (the thoracic wall), intercostal muscles (between the ribs), and the diaphragm, the most important muscle involved in breathing.

@ *The Process of Breathing*

As you inhale, the diaphragm lowers and the ribs rise. In exhalation the reverse occurs.This cycle of inhalation and exhalation occurs about eighteen times per minute when the body is at rest. The rhythmic expansion and contraction of the diaphragm affects the whole person. Efficient and balanced breathing patterns will positively affect your mental, emotional, and physical well-being so it is important to focus on breathing properly. Using Shamanic massage can open and help clear the respiratory system and support efficient breathing. The trachea or lungs can sometimes be blocked by particles that inhibit the proper action of the system. By clearing the respiratory system, Shamanic massage helps strengthen breathing and the system gains energy.

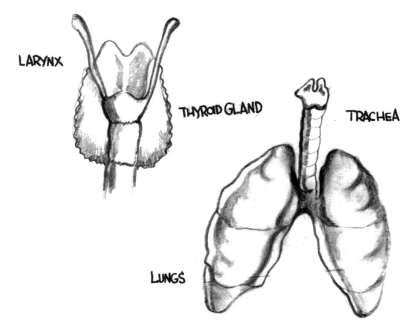

The Respiratory System.

@ Shamanic Massage Benefits the Respiratory System by:

- Improving breathing patterns.
- Assisting relief of chronic respiratory difficulties such as asthma and bronchitis.

THE DIGESTIVE SYSTEM

The digestive system breaks food into chemical components that can be used by the body for energy and cell restoration. The digestive system includes the mouth, salivary glands, pharynx, esophagus, stomach, large and small intestines, pancreas, liver, gallbladder, and appendix. The tube-like structure of it runs through the body and is known as the alimentary canal.

Food passes from the mouth, where it is prepared for digestion by chewing and ensalivation, through the pharynx and esophagus to the stomach, where it it is held while stomach acid breaks it down further. Within three to four hours of eating, the stomach is empty and digestion continues in the small intestine by means of bile (secreted by the liver), pancreatic juice, and intestinal juice.

The liver is responsible for purifying the body and producing new cells. Many believe it ranks in importance with the heart in maintaining a strong, healthy body. Massaging the internal organs can release stored emotional trauma, relieve gas, and in some cases even soothe pain in this area. Pressing acupressure points and massaging the colon and the stomach can also bring relief to various digestive disorders.

◉ Benefits of Shaman Massage for the Digestive System

- Improving liver function.
- Relieving spastic colon.
- Acting as a mechanical cleanser, pushing out waste products, particularly in those who suffer from constipation.

THE URINARY SYSTEM

The main functions of the urinary system are elimination of waste from the body, maintenance of the body's water balance. The principal organs are the kidneys, ureters, bladder, and urethra. Urine is secreted by the kidneys through the ureters to the bladder, stored in the bladder, and then is discharged through the urethra. Physicians and healers analyze urine to aid in detecting diseases of the kidney and other parts of the urinary tract. At least one kidney must function in order for life to be sustained.

◉ Benefits of Shaman Massage for the Urinary System

- Cleanse the blood and balance water element.
- In cases of abnormal swelling in the body, bodywork can affect the elimination of fluids.

THE ROLE OF ANATOMY AND PHYSIOLOGY IN HEALING

You do not have to know the names of all the bones, muscles and nerves to give a good Shaman massage. When body manipulation is used for even the most general therapeutic purposes, such as releasing tight muscles or relieving tension, a basic understanding of how the body/mind elements interface and how massage affects the body's various organs and systems will help you in several important ways. First, you will be better able to gauge which bodywork techniques are best. Second, you can begin to relate common special symptoms to particular bodywork techniques that may be helpful. Most important, an understanding of how your own body works will aid you in your overall health regimen.

Healing touch is an essential part of that regimen; the essence of any bodywork is intuitive, hands-on, communicative contact.

HEALING HANDS AND SHAMAN MASSAGE TECHNIQUES

@ Pull and Stretch Traction

This is a fairly simple technique applied to the legs.

Step 1
While your partner is lying on his or her back, grasp one of your partner's feet in each hand.

Step 2
Holding them firmly, slowly and steadily lean all your body weight backward.

Step 3
This should give a good stretch to your partner's hip and lower back muscles.

Caution: Avoid using this technique on people suffering from osteoporosis or other bone disorders. Also be sensitive to those who have recently had hip, knee, or ankle injuries.

@ Increasing Joint Motion

This is a gentle movement to help evaluate areas requiring healing and to improve flexibility in the joints. You can evaluate certain factors in a person's emotional life by the condition of the muscles associated with each joint. By working each joint through its range of motion you can release emotional holding points while reducing muscular tension.

Step 1
Slowly rotate the joint through its normal range of motion. Move it in all directions including clockwise and counterclockwise. Hold the body part to be worked on in your hand to give it support as you move the joint.

Step 2
Tightness or limitation in movement can sometimes be relieved by gently shaking the limb and then moving it through range of motion. If this does not reduce stiffness, apply pressure on the point of stiffness.

Step 3
Repeat gentle joint mobilization exercises periodically—about every two or three hours—until the tightness or limitation of movement is lessened. Slowly rotate the joints three times in one direction and then three times in the opposite direction. Repeat this cycle three times.

@ Circular Pressure Point Massage

This technique is similar to Rhythmic Pressure Point Massage but requires a rhythmic circular motion rather than an up-down pressure. This is the technique to choose for muscle spasms or cramps and is one of the main techniques for healing damaged tissue and reducing the formation of scar tissue after surgery or sprains. It can be done very lightly or with firm pressure. I usually define the the amount of pressure I use by the terms "gentle," "firm," or "deep," but the amount of pressure used will depend on your partner's tolerance for pain. Whichever pressure is used, the approach is the same.

CHAPTER 5

@

AROMATHERAPY AND HERBAL HEALING

@ What Is Aromatherapy?

Aromatherapy is the use of essential oils extracted from the flower, leaf, stalk or fruit of a plant, shrub or tree to revitalize and enhance both physical, mental, emotional and spiritual health. We all experience a simple form of emotional healing with aromatherapy in our daily lives when we peel an orange, wash our face with a mint-scented soap, or wear a carnation in our lapel.

The term "essential" refers to the fact that the plant liquid has been refined to the point where all impurities have been removed and nothing but wholesome and healing elements remain.

Essential oils are hormones, regulators, and catalysts which exist in tiny droplets between the cells of the plant. They are extracted by one of several different methods: with chemical solvents, by cold expression or by steam distillation.

An individual who is interested in exploring the Shamanic process can access an altered state of consciousness through aromatic oils. There are four key physical responses that the human body has when presented with a powerful or intense "aroma":

1. Gagging or heaving. This can be a response to unpleasant, rotten or offensive food, or to aromas that remind one of unpleasant memories.

2. A sense of pleasure and relaxation, associated with a feeling of being safe or nurtured.

3. The intense physical response that people exhibit when they

feel assaulted by an aroma such as a strong cheese, cigar smoke, hospital antiseptic, or alcohol on someone's breath.

4. The sexual arousal that comes when an individual associates a scent with a person or memory.

Aromatic oils are a powerful means for creating responses, both chemically and emotionally. The basic process involves the use of various plant and flower derived scents and aromas. Each of these is drawn into the body in such a way as to alter physiology and mood and to influence psychological and spiritual states. Aromatherapy is healing to the emotions because it helps us to experience our feelings more deeply and opens the doors to new realities.

@ *Your Sense of Smell*

The ability to smell is among the most subtle and expansive of all the senses. The sense of smell is humbling in its complexity. While the visual system can create thousands of hues out of just three color receptors—one tuned to red, another to blue, and a third to green—and the tongue can distinguish a few variables— sweet, sour, bitter, and salty—the thousand or so distinct odor receptors located in the nerve tissue of the nasal cavity in mammals can distinguish over 10,000 odors. Although the sense of smell is complex, it is also the most basic, primal, and intimate of senses.

In the Shamanic process, smell connects us to our essential, primal nature, for even in most animals it is the sense of smell that dominates. Throughout nature it is the ability to smell that enables animals to find food or a mate. People can survive with the loss of sight, hearing or smell, and yet so much that affects us emotionally is tied to smell.

@ *The Scientific Connection*

Without smell an infant would be unable to locate its mother's nipple. Studies have shown that a mother can pick out her own newborn through the sense of smell. How is this possible? Research- ers disclosed in 1991 that they had located protein-based odor recep- tors that wind through the membranes of sensory nerves found in a small patch of tissue (the olfactory epithelium). This tissue patch is located directly behind the bridge of the nose. It is thought that when a person is breathing in a scent or chewing or swallowing, an odor molecule is pushed upward and rises through the air to meet the membrane receptor in the nose. This receptor changes shape and, as a result, the quality of the nerve cell is altered. That change stimulates the nerve to send a smell signal toward the brain.

The connection between the sense of smell and the brain is a fascinating study in the workings of nature. Researchers have found that many of the nerves involved in smelling extend some of their axons directly into the part of the brain that is the seat of sexuality, drive and the emotions. Known as the limbic system of the brain, this neurological route of smell is much more direct than that taken by auditory or visual input.

◉ Our Tribal Sense of Smell

Many of our responses to various smells are based on our beliefs. What may smell foul in one culture may seem pleasant in another. There are few smells that create the same response in all peoples. A flower that smells sweet in one culture, may be associated with death in another.

I know many city people who, when driving on a highway or walking through the woods, find a slight skunk odor to be a pleasant experience because they associate it with being in a rural environment. The line between the smell of skunk, civet and musk is a thin one, and yet skunk is often associated with unpleasant qualities, while civet and musk are ingredients in expensive perfumes. The former is found near the anus of the African civet cat while musk was originally isolated from glands in the abdomen of the male musk deer.

◉ How Are Aromatic Oils Used?

In order to use essential oils effectively it is important to understand their history as well as what these oils are and where they come from.

"Aromatherapy," the practice of using oils to heal, dates back at least to ancient Egyptian times, when a multitude of essential oils and aromatic substances were used at every step of the very complex, sophisticated—and effective—process of embalming for mummification. The use of these oils in the West can be traced through ancient Greece, Rome, the Middle Ages through the Renaissance and all the way to the present time. Their general use in holistic health practices, as well as their use in Shamanic practices throughout Asia and Africa, is well documented.

@ Extracting These Oils?

The most effective method for extracting aromatic oils from plants without loss of potency and vibrational integrity is through steam distillation. Fresh plant parts are placed in a vessel and subjected to a powerful "steam bath." The moisture and intense heat of the steam drives the oils out of the organic material, which results in a liquid condensate. The oils are then skimmed off the surface of the resulting solution, leaving a water-soluble plant extract. Scientists call this solution hydrosol. Some oils cannot be extracted easily through steam distillation. For example citrus essences are usually expeller-pressed (removed under pressure) from the peels, as citrus rind is too tough and thick to respond well to the steaming process.

In another approach to oil extraction, flower essences are collected by mixing petals with a solvent such as ethyl alcohol, which is then filtered and evaporated at reduced pressure, leaving behind what is often called an "absolute." Several procedures may be performed on essential oils after extraction. Oils such as eucalyptus can be redistilled or rectified, for instance, which removes many non-essential elements which are not eliminated by the initial extraction. An essential oil is often extended with alcohol which can alter its aroma and effect. Most of the oils sold in pharmacies and produced by large pharmaceutical companies are chemically extracted. This is frowned on by most serious herbalists, the belief being that this form of extraction lowers the vibrational quality of the oils.

@ Ways Aromatic Oils Are Used?

Aromatherapy usually involves the use of plant essences in four ways:

1. Through aromatherapy baths.
2. Through inhalation of the scents given off by oils.
3. Through direct inhalation of the scents given off by simmering flowers, herbs, spices and other plants in water.
4. Through Shaman massage using aromatic oils.

Note: Not all aromatic oils can be utilized in the same manner. In fact some can be dangerous if used improperly:

1. Never ingest an aromatic oil unless you are absolutely sure it is not dangerous or poisonous.
2. Be aware that some people can have strong allergic reactions to certain oils.
3. Some oils may be too strong to apply directly to the skin and can cause severe skin reactions.

@ What Types of Oils Are Best?

Many aromatic oils that are available at flea markets or in perfume stores are made from synthetic ingredients and are not acceptable as an effective healing tool. Many Shamanic practitioners believe that it is critical to know how to distinguish a plant-derived oil from an imitation. Artificial oils that mimic the scent of natural fragrances have no therapeutic value, and it is the spirit connection between the practitioner and the plants that is the key in the Shamanic process. Synthetic oils have low or weak Chi (life energy). Plants which produce authentic essences can synthesize in a way human ingenuity cannot begin to comprehend. These plant-produced oils absorb natural forces present in sunlight, rain, soil and air.

Many oils which are advertised as essential are, in fact, completely synthetic. Synthetic oils are petrochemical derivatives which, besides contributing to environmental destruction, are linked to countless cases of chemical sensitivity.

By contrast, perfumers blending pure essential oils during the plagues of the Middle Ages were among the few healthy survivors. Aromatics were burned in buildings to fumigate them from infestations. In one documented instance, burning juniper prevented the population of an entire town from being stricken by a plague that ravished the entire surrounding area.

It is worth noting here that the FDA requires only that ingredients used for scent in personal care products—shampoo, hand lotion, perfume, etc.—be listed as "fragrance." Unless the manufacturer states that the fragrance is "essential oil," it is impossible to determine what it contains. Estimates are that of all fragrances claiming to be pure, about 90 percent are not pure.

Some suppliers have slyly expanded their definition of essential oils to include oils that match the molecular configurations of essential oil as defined in the specifications of the Essential Oil Congress. So-called "nature identicals" are derived from petrochemicals and diluted with over 80 percent alcohol, which is denatured with diethyl phthalate or brucine sulfate.

Another common misconception concerns certain flowers whose essences are not extractable. For example: magnolia, honeysuckle, lilac, carnation, violet and gardenia. If you see these in a product or a perfume, or sold as an essential oil, you know immediately that they are made from petrochemicals and not from flowers.

In addition, scents derived from animals, such as musk and ambergris, besides being prohibitively expensive and, in some cases, illegal, do not belong in botanical blends.

@ *Recognizing Plant-Derived Essential Oils:*

When choosing an acceptable oil, look for products that:

- Are thin and watery and evaporate easily.
- Do not leave a grease mark on paper once evaporated.
- Have an overpoweringly strong scent.

@ *Creating Your Own Healing Formulas*

Essential oils oils work synergistically. That is, they complement and enhance each other's properties when mixed. For this reason, it is usually best to blend between two and four oils of desired properties and with aromas pleasing to the user. Once you mix more than four oils together, the mixture will be powerful in a new way but the strength of the individual oils will be reduced.

It is difficult to use undiluted aromatic oils in massage since they have a very strong scent and evaporate at room temperature. The friction that takes place during massage causes them to evaporate even faster. For this reason it is best to mix the aromatic oils with a liquid carrier oil or fixed oil. These oils are lubricating and protect the skin from the abrasion of a strong massage. They are also valuable in aromatherapy massage because they hold the essential oils longer so that they may be absorbed by the skin rather than just evaporating. Carrier oils must be of vegetable origin and fine textured, with little or no smell. Apricot kernel, almond, canola, evening primrose, grape seed, safflower, and sunflower oils are best. Avocado, olive and wheat germ are much thicker, and are best mixed with the lighter carrier oils just mentioned.

When preparing your formulas remember that the correct ratio of essential oil to carrier oil is generally six drops to two teaspoons. These precious healing oils, like all herbal products, should always be stored in tightly closed, dark glass bottles to prevent deterioration of their healing properties. Add a few drops of vitamin E to extend oil potency.

@ Caution

A word about the power of essential oils. Though they are taken orally in many Shamanic practices, the program described in this book focuses on the external use of plant oils. Herbs may be dangerous if used over a long period of time, as can be many of the oils that are derived from them. If you choose to explore aromatic oils outside the realm described here, I strongly recommend that you find a skilled herbalist to supervise your studies.

Some people may have an allergic reaction or sensitivity to some oils. Before mixing oils for massage it is wise to place a small amount of oil on a sensitive area of the skin as a test.

@ Aromatherapy Can Be Employed in a Number of Different Ways:

- **Bath.** When added to a bath, oils of lavendar, marjoram, chamomile, hyssop and rosemary can work to stimulate skin, relax tense, sore muscles, and relieve headache, fatigue and nervous tension.
- **Compress.** For bruises, aches and pains and irritated skin, a compress of birch, chamomile, juniper, rosemary, nutmeg, thyme or vetiver can be helpful.
- **Friction Chest Rub.** Mix the essence in a base of lanolin and cocoa butter. Then rub the compound on your chest morning and night.
- **Inhalation.** Sprinkle 6 to 8 drops of essence on a tissue. Inhale deeply three times. Caution: Close eyes when inhaling.
- **Shaman Massage.** One of the most popular ways to use aromatherapy oils is in massage. Oils like coriander, vertivert, cinnamon, ylang-ylang and neroli are a few of many which work to

improve circulation and relax the nervous system. This is an effective way of using amber. Amber is a crystallized mixture of resins native to India, and is considered the King of Scents. The unique fragrance of amber is spiritually enlivening, sensual, pleasing, and has a focusing effect on the mind. The best way to use amber is to rub it on your skin or clothing.

◉ Spiritual Aromatherapy

Different oils and resins are noted for the quality they have to create a spiritually centered environment. Sage is burned to clean an area of weak or unbalanced psychic energy. Sandalwood oil is used to create a meditative environment in many Shamanic traditions.

My favorite oil for lifting the spirit has always been camphor. Camphor is a white crystalline substance obtained from special cinnamon trees of India and Sri Lanka. These trees grow very slowly and camphor cannot be removed until a tree is 50 years old. Camphor is one of the most Shamanically oriented of the aromatic healing tools. Known through recorded history for its calming effect, it was commonly used to treat colds and was valuable for so many different ailments that it became known as the "balsam of disease." Throughout Asia, camphor is valued by everyone, from the poorest to the wealthiest. Camphor burns readily, and in some Hindu temples small tablets are ignited and used in ceremonial fires. This is to symbolize the burning away of all traces of negative karma. In certain yogic schools, camphor is used to support celibacy. Yogis found that camphor had a calming effect on the system and as a whole would relieve irritations to the sexual organs. Much of the camphor available in the West comes from India and can be purchased in pellet form.

◉ How to Use Aromatic Oils

Orally. (Use only under professional supervision.) Place about eight drops of each oil in a glass of lukewarm water. Be sure to combine no more than three or four oils and use no more than 25 to 40 drops of all ingredients combined. Take the mixture 10 minutes before meals three times a day. For children, limit the dosage to 3 to 10 drops three times a day.

Note: Essential oils evaporate quickly when added to warm water and so must be used immediately. Also, some essences are too powerful to be taken orally. Consult a qualified specialist.

@ Room Dispersal

An essence can be effectively dispersed throughout a room by use of an atomizer. Another good method is to buy a small heat lamp with a crucible. The heat vaporizes the essence and disperses it throughout the room. Heat lamps are available at many stores that sell essences. A good source for aromatic oils and dispersal equipment is: Aroma Vera, P.O. Box 3609, Culver City, CA 90231; (213) 675-8219.

@ Steaming

Steaming with essential oils can be an effective deep cleansing treatment for the delicate skin of the face. Inhaling the aroma of benzoin, eucalyptus, pine and spruce can relieve sinus congestion resulting from the common cold.

Add three or four drops of essence to a basin of hot water. Lean over the basin with a towel over your head to trap the vapors and inhale deeply several times.

Caution: Not to be used by persons suffering from asthma. Concentrated steam may cause choking.

@ Topically

Many essences are concentrated. Therefore, rather than apply them full strength, soak a compress in a diluted essence twice a day and apply to the afflicted area.

HOW DEBRA R. REDUCED HER STRESS

About twenty years ago, I met Debra R., a very pleasant woman who had been going from doctor to doctor for the treatment of various health problems. She suffered from sexual problems, insomnia, and fatigue. She was only 48 years old, yet she was one of the saddest and most overwhelmed people I had ever met in my life.

When I met her she had tears in her eyes. Whenever one condition seemed to improve, another one would come to take its place. Her headaches had only recently subsided when suddenly every joint in her body became swollen, hot and painful.

I had no idea how to help her other than to investigate her general life-style and emotional health. I soon learned that she was in a constant state of stress. She had two jobs and spent weekends taking care of her elderly father. She had few friends, never exercised, never took vacations or even took the time to read a book, watch a movie or a television show. She was always running from one responsibility to another or solving one crisis and then running to solve the next. She was completely overwhelmed by stress.

She seemed utterly helpless and yet I knew I could help her. I knew that trying to eliminate all of her stress and tension was both impractical and impossible, but there was certainly one way to minimize their effects: aromatherapy. She said that she loved perfumes and the smell of fresh flowers and was willing to try aromatherapy if I thought it might help.

@ The Steps Taken to Reduce Debra's Stress Were as Follows:

1. Whenever she felt deep anxiety, depression, or apathy, she took a bath with Patchouli Oil.
2. I recommended that she avoid eating meals in a stressed-out state. She began inhaling frankincense just before eating lunch. This relaxed her while at the same time stimulating her mind, as well as her digestion.
3. Meditation. When Debra became overstressed she would sit for a few minutes, taking long slow deep breaths of rose oil and thinking about nothing at all. This helped calm her down.
4. Debra carried small bottles of lavender and geranium oil that she had purchased in a health food store. When she became stressed and could not meditate, she would impregnate absorbent cotton with these oils and inhale deeply or, if possible, take a warm bath and add a few drops of these oils to the bath water.

   Debra's relief was rapid and dramatic. Her depression diminished and then disappeared. One by one her health problems abated. She was amazed. It seemed that all of her conditions were the result of stress. Her life-style had prevented her from responding to each new emotional and physical crisis. Aromatherapy had freed her. Now she was well.

@ General Healing Herbs

In addition to healing oils many Shamanic healers make teas and extracts from plants. Ancient Egyptian and Chinese texts thousands of years old have recorded the use of herbs for treating and curing various ailments of the body, mind and spirit.

Many of the plants used today in herbal medicine were used and described by Dioscorides, a first-century Greek physician and botanist who wrote a reference work on botany and the therapeutic use of plants.

The use of herbal teas, extracts and powders to help rebuild sickly and weak bodies is still used by virtually every culture. Many Native American communities used herbs for medicine, dyes, poisons and food. The Aztecs used nettles regularly and early American pioneers used lovage, sage, chives, lily of the valley, peppermint, thyme, flax, pennyroyal and chamomile. The English used dandelion and the Chinese, ginseng.

Today many herbs are used in modern medicine. Though the operation of many herbal remedies is not fully understood, they are the basis of some well known pharmaceuticals. It was the cinchona tree that gave us quinine for the treatment of malaria, the foxglove plant that gave us digitalis. Other herbs that are currently used by medical doctors in one form or another include red periwinkle, mayapple, witch hazel, cayenne pepper, gingko, garlic and ginseng. St.-John's-wort is used to reduce depression.

Though there is more sophisticated research on the value of herbal medicines than ever before, most of the information about herbs used in natural healing is based on the folklore passed down from generation to generation. Over the last fifteen years the use of herbal medicines in healing has increased to an amazing level. Herbal experts cite these major reasons why herbs have gained new found popularity:

1) many people desire to return to nature;
2) they fear the side effects associated with many over-the-counter and prescription drugs;
3) they are unhappy with the high cost and impersonal style of orthodox medicine;

4) they've discovered that Indian, African, Asian, and South American cultures have used herbal medicines with great success.

@ Why Are Herbal Medicines Sometimes the Center of Controversy

Many of the negative associations that medical doctors harbor toward herbal medicine are based on the fact that many commercially available herbal products are of poor quality. Some products do not even contain any of the herbs that are listed on the labels. This is especially true with ginseng formulas. To remedy this, many herb companies have formed trade associations in an attempt to upgrade the quality of their products.

As valuable as herbs are to the natural healing process, it is foolish to make believe that all herbal substances are free from danger. Many herbs contain deadly poisons, toxic substances or powerful alkaloids. Herbs that may be of great medicinal value may be poisonous if used improperly and thus should never be used except under the guidance of a well-trained herbalist or a physician who has a strong working knowledge of herbal medicine. Many safe formulas can be purchased in natural food stores as tea or in extract form.

@ Make Your Own Herbal Oils

Making your own herbal oils is easy and is especially powerful in Shamanic healing since your own energy infuses into the energy field of the plants. These oils are used differently from the way highly concentrated essential oils are used, and they are extracted differently as well. Three of my favorite oils are marigold (calendula), eucalyptus and peppermint. Calendula oil is soothing to skin irritations. Rubbing eucalyptus and peppermint oil into the skin can help relieve aching muscles.

@ How to Prepare an Herbal Oil

1. Gather fresh herbs and pack them up to the top of a clear glass pint jar.
2. Using extra-virgin olive oil or sweet almond oil, fill the jar till the herbs are completely covered. Placing a tablespoon of rubbing alcohol on top will prevent mold growth.

3. With the top covered, place the jar in a dry, sunny, spot for about ten to fourteen days. Shake daily.

4. Using cheesecloth that you can obtain at any hardware store, strain the oil and store it in a cool dark place. The jar should be tightly covered. This oil will be good to use for three or four months.

INTERMEDIATE HANDS-ON HEALING TECHNIQUES

@ *Gravity Rocking*

This very gentle technique is used to release surface tension and superficial energy blocks in the body and to stimulate the sensory motor nerves, thus readying the body for other techniques. Muscle Rock is excellent for removing both emotional and physical tension and consequently is a very good way to prepare the body for a complete Shaman Massage session. It is a technique that strongly mimics the rocking motion that a mother might use in soothing a child.

Step 1
Place the palm of your hand on the muscle to be rocked where there is tension or discomfort. Use a very gentle touch with no pressure. Wrap your fingers around the muscle so that the palm and fingers are touching the body. Rest your free hand on the joint above the area to be rocked. For example, for rocking the front thighs, rest the upper hand on the pelvic bone. If rocking the lower arm, rest the hand on the elbow joint. If rocking the buttocks, rest the upper hand on the back.

Step 2
With your hand resting firmly on the body part, slowly start to rock your palm back and forth in a firm, but non-forced movement. You can move your palm either horizontally or vertically. Rock for about two minutes.

Step 3
Placing yourself on the right side of your partner with your right hand resting gently on their abdomen and your left hand gently on their forehead, slowly start to rock your palm back and forth

in a gentle, non-forced movement. You can move your right palm either horizontally or vertically. Rock for about two minutes. Do not rock the hand that is resting on your partner's forehead.

Gravity Rocking is a very soothing technique that seems to create a sense of tranquility between the giver and the receiver in much the same way that a mother's rocking has a soothing effect on both the mother and baby. It is valuable for those in a state of fear or terror.

Note: Make certain that your palm does not slide around (no lubricant is used). Do not grab, pinch, or press on the muscle.

@ *The Muscle Hug*

This technique is used when a muscle is tight, flaccid, or weak. Its purpose is to bring strength and tone to the muscle. Although this technique is performed most easily on the legs, arms, and head, it can be done on any muscles. This technique should be applied on the bare skin since it is not very effective when done through clothing. It is most effective when used on the buttocks, the upper and lower arms, and the upper and lower legs.

Step 1
Place one hand on either end of the muscle, near the surrounding joints. This technique is always applied between two joints. For example, on the thigh, place your hands firmly on the muscles that lie between the hip joint and the knee. Grasp the muscle firmly (but not so hard as to cause pain or discomfort) with your entire hand. Be careful not to dig into the muscle with your nails.

Step 2
With your hands around the muscle, firmly but gently press hands toward one another, then pull away so that that muscle is first manually contracted and then stretched.

If you are holding the muscle properly, friction and chafing will not take place.

Step 3
Repeat contraction and stretching ten times.

CHAPTER 6

@

THE VISION QUEST

ALTERED STATES

Many people who are interested in Shamanism are confused by the concept of altered states of consciousness and non-ordinary reality. You have experienced an altered state of consciousness if you have ever day dreamed or driven a car "on automatic pilot." Do you remember the time where your mind seemed to wander somewhere else and yet the car drove safely for miles, even getting off at the correct exit? There is no single defining factor of what this state consists of; however, there are various recognizable factors that indicate that a person has entered it.

1. There is a sense of egolessness. It is as if a person feels as if they are merging with people and objects around them. As if they are in a single state of consciousness.
2. A distorted sense of time and space. There is a breakdown of normal boundaries. Intuition takes over in situations where a rational approach was the normal operating model.
3. Extraordinary psychic and other mental powers.
4. An intense and accurate sensitivity to the emotional states of others.
5. A trance-like state, often called the state of flow.

Because a Shamanic state is generally noted through external observation, it is difficult to measure it with the traditional tools of empirical science. As mathematics and physics have integrated more and more theoretical ideas into rational theory the mystic sciences have filtered into Western academic thought.

@ The State of Flow

In a state of flow, you feel as if you have actually become one with the activity you are focused on. You may lose track of your body, emotions, sense of time and even of your physical location. When you are giving everything you can to a particular vision or challenge, you become free of fear and anxiety. You have no room in your consciousness for boredom. Many people I have spoken with who function in this way speak of it as a "drug-free high" that comes from the rhythm that seems to be part and parcel of working at this 100% level. Many people relate to this when they drive a car. There is an "automatic pilot" effect. You know where you are going, and you are driving effectively and safely, and yet your mind is not intensely focused on the road. One is still paying attention to detail and focusing, but the state is different from intense concentration. It is not the type of concentration that creates great mental strain. The easiest way to describe "state of flow" is that you function at a level of excellence with ease.

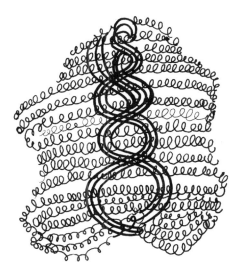

"Chi" and The Vision Quest. Based on a chart on Page 191 Polarity Therapy, Vol. 2, by Dr. Randolph Stone.

🌀 How the State of Flow Works

Dr. Mike Csikszentmihalyi, a respected behavioral scientist at the University of Chicago, has indicated that the state of flow involves a sensitive balance between specific skills that an individual possesses and the challenges that these skills must be applied to. If the challenge is too basic, we may become bored. If the challenge, on the other hand, is way beyond the skills that are available to us, we may become distressed and fearful, and avoid addressing the challenge at all. When you are in a state of flow, you are in essence rowing along a gentle, smooth-flowing stream as opposed to trying to row a boat up a waterfall. Through the Vision Quest and the Hands-On Healing this altered state called "state of flow" becomes available to each person.

🌀 There Are Two Types of Altered States

Research done in sensory deprivation units (flotation tanks) has found that there are generally two types of altered states.

1. Quieting of the mind: This is the state achieved in prayer, meditation, and deep visualization, Hands-On Healing and Shamanic Massage.

2. Intense stimulation of the mind and senses: This usually done through internal and external sensory or intellectual overload: This can include extremes as varied as intellectual mulling over a Zen Koan (a philosophical paradox used to break down attachment to the rational mind), the use of psychoactive drugs, Hands-On Healing and Shamanic Massage, terror, fasting (food deprivation), sleep deprivation, a life challenging event, extreme sports, and extreme physical or emotional pain.

These two states are not mutually exclusive since they may merge and flow through each other, just as the black and white of the Yin-Yang symbol in Taoism melt into each other.

The definition of mental illness as opposed to the Shamanic state can be complex. One of my teachers once told me with a chuckle that the line between a Shaman and a person with mental illness can loosely be noted in that the Shaman never answers inner voices in public, whereas one tortured by mental illness would do so. The Shamanic altered state can create a sense of "Ecstasy."

This word is derived from Greek words that mean "to stand outside oneself." A person doing a Hands-On Healing session often feels as if they are outside themselves. It is a tranquil, intense, healing experience. It is a state of Ecstasy.

While scientists still struggle with the idea of the problem of consciousness, exploring where the body/mind connection begins or ends, there is a revolution taking place. It is a conscious revolution of transformation. Hands-On Healing is a vehicle for this revolution.

◉ Are You Ready to Begin Your Vision Quest?

A Vision Quest is a journey into personal inquiry. If you review the things in life that you may desire or that you have already accomplished or achieved, you may be surprised. Many of us define what we want not by the concept of gaining something but rather by avoiding something. Even people of great wealth may have achieved such wealth out of the desire to avoid poverty. Many people strive to have what they see as great power because they were raised in an environment where they felt powerless. In order to truly achieve something that you desire and be able to enjoy that achievement in a joyous and fearless manner, it is essential that you create a proactive vision, one where your actions and thoughts are based on magnificent possibilities, not what you wish to avoid. To do otherwise is to be at the mercy of circumstance.

During the Vision Quest you are timeless. You aren't looking behind you nor in front of you. You are in the moment, seeing clearly where you are right here and now. At that moment you are on the journey. To begin the Vision Quest there are certain sacred steps you take:

1. Create or access a "sacred place." A Sacred Place is a physical or psychological retreat that you enter for guidance and relaxation.
2. Begin a personal training program in creative visualization. This is a tool for integrating mind and body. Through visualization you become clear, focused, relaxed and stress free.
3. Develop visualization skills for healing. These are specific visualizations whose purpose it is to eliminate psychological and physical pain and discomfort.
4. Develop your intuitive skills. Intuition is more than just a gut feeling about something. For those properly trained it is the door-

way for angels, spirit guides and all manner of Shamanic messengers to speak to you.

5. Hands-On Healing and Personal Transformation. This involves integrating 14 key affirmations that relate to each of the Shaman Massage Techniques. When you repeat any of these affirmations before your Hands-On Healing Session and repeat them throughout the session, they will begin to free you from your personal obstacles and give you the means to move past them. This clarity balances your own Chi and expands the power in your Hands-On Healing session. In a sense you are receiving a healing session at the same time that you are giving one, and the one you are giving becomes wondrous.

THE FIRST STEP ON THE VISION QUEST

@ Creating Your Sacred Place

A Sacred Place is a central element of the Vision Quest. A sacred place may be indoors or out. When it cannot be created psychically it can be symbolized through language and visual imagery. It is a place where you are in the world but not of it. It is a place where you detach your attention from sensory stimulation and turn inward. In this environment your intuition can come to the surface and your angels and spirit guides can make themselves known. Here are some steps you can take to create a physical sacred place:

1. Create a sacred place that has a private place of entry.
2. Make it quiet, safe and comfortable.
3. Create a sense of sensory separation from your normal environment. Fill your place with sensuous detail. Use Power objects: incense, candles, aromatic oils, amber.
4. Allow a physical and psychological space for your inner guide or another person to comfortably be with you.

@ Physical Places

If you live in the city, a sacred place can be a quiet lobby of a building that is rich in fine architectural detail. Some cities have public, indoor spaces with waterfalls or pleasant music. Find a place in such a space that intuitively feels ''like home.''

If you live in the country your sacred place may be a private lookout point over a valley or at the foot of a mountain, a path next to a pond or near a waterfall.

@ *Visualization*

Visualization is a form of mental sense impression. For many years Shamanic practitioners have used inspiration, communication and visualization skills in combination to rapidly increase individual awareness and effectiveness. By using visual imagery, these practitioners have found that their students become more emotionally and physically receptive and that the benefits are recognizable almost immediately. The beneficial response to visualization techniques has been especially pronounced for individuals involved with stress management programs.

When reading articles about people who have made a difference in the world, you will notice that they often had a vision at the very beginning of their journey that made them confident of the successes to come. The evident power of visualization reinforces the concept that there is a direct relationship between the health of the body and the mind. When a person is in a balanced state of health, their life objectives and visions will be more clearly defined. With this clarity of thought and focus, the ability arises to act with greater effectiveness. This is so because with this clarity comes the knowledge that positive results are just around the corner.

Mental imagery and visualization play vital roles in all aspects of personal development both in the early creative and innovative phase and in later phases when innovation is applied through action. In the articles and books about imagery and visualization there is one fundamental point: As you think, so will you become.

PREPARING YOURSELF FOR UNLIMITED POSSIBILITIES

- Choose a time of day that you believe will be most creative for you.
- Write your vision down on paper.
  a. Specify it.
  b. Create various physical scenarios it might appear as.
  c. Inquire: That means putting it in the form of a question that requires more than one answer.

- At first you should work on this project alone.
- Cut off interruptions; they can stop the flow of your creative juices. Don't answer phones, don't get snacks, etc.
- True creativity does not have to make sense. Ask yourself, "In what way can this project be improved, changed, or modified in any way, whether it seems rational, reasonable, possible, probable or sensible, etc."

Types of Visualization

You may not realize it but we all visualize throughout the day. When you remember something from the past, have daydreams, or have a quiet conversation with yourself, you are visualizing. In the Shamanic process, you will harness your visualizations and consciously employ them for healing and self-knowledge. Visualizations can help you to consciously train your body to short circuit stress through relaxation.

There Are Three Forms of Visualization:

1. Inquiry Visualization: Create a visual image of an ocean beach or a mountaintop, some pleasant nature scene. As this scene brings you a sense of freedom and relaxation, free your mind of any thoughts for about ten seconds. Now ask a question relating to your own healing or spiritual growth. Begin the question with any of the following words, "who, what, where, when, how, which?" An example would be, "What do I need to do now to be content?" Now wait for an answer to the question. Many Shamans teach that the truth lies within you. The response to your question may arise from your subconscious to your consciousness.

An Inquiry Visualization Exercise

It is vital that you identify those domains where you need more information to assure the completion of the vision quest. The following questions will help you identify these areas:

1. What is a personal strength I have which, if effectively applied, will fulfill my vision?
2. What steps, if neglected, will most likely create unnecessary struggle?

3. What details will require my focused and continuous attention to assure achievement of my vision?
4. How should I commit my time to the various goals which, when combined, will fulfill my vision quest?
5. Am I focusing on details at the expense of innovation and creative activity?
6. Do I create physical and spiritual support wherever possible?

2. Creative visualization: This the most common of the various types of visualization. Creative visualization uses all of the memory senses: taste, smell, sight, and sound. This is a technique used by everyone from high-school athletes to successful businesspeople. In this technique, one imagines a goal that one wants to attain. This might be a world record or an acceleration in healing and wellness.

@ *A Creative Visualization Exercise*

Once you have defined your vision then it is time to look at the details. Again it is important to remember that asking questions is the way to go.

1. What are the benefits?
2. How long will it last?
3. Is there a less expensive way?
4. How will a support team make it easier?
5. Is there a more effective way?
6. How can it be modified?
7. Could it be adapted to different uses?
8. What can be rearranged? subtracted? substituted? added? combined? reversed?

3. Guided Visualization: This is a combination of elements found in inquiry visualization and creative visualization. In this technique you actively visualize some scene or process, but you have no end goal. You might imagine yourself walking along a path in the woods. You can sense the trees, hear the sound of the leaves. Walking along you come to a waterfall. There is a path behind the waterfall that leads to a tunnel with a beautiful purple or violet light at the end of it. You walk into the tunnel.

Notice that in this visualization you are in touch with the details but there is no apparent end to the visualization. In this process you are creating an environment where your inner guides can supply the missing pieces in your quest.

Remember: The intention of all our visualizations is to create a healing bond between body, mind and spirit and create an open space for your inner guides to manifest. In the early stages of your Shamanic development inner guides will connect to you through your intuition.

@ Preparing for the Visualization Experience

1. Wear loose clothing, lie down or sit in a comfortable chair, preferably in a quiet place.
2. Scan your body from head to toe. Focus on any specific areas that seem tight.
3. Visualize that you are taking a long full breath into the area that is tense, and exhale the tension.
4. If the area does not relax, create a visual image of the tension or pain and use a relaxing image to facilitate the release process.
5. Once the body feels completely relaxed, create a mental experience of all of your senses: hearing, sight, smell, taste and touch. Imagine a sound, possibly trees rustling in the wind. Now imagine that you see the trees that are making those sounds, smell the flowers or leaves on the tree, taste the berries, feel the bark. Expand to the sound of birds, the forest, the sky above the forest, the sound of your feet walking past the tree, the waterfall in the distance.
6. Repeat one of the 18 affirmations listed for The Hands-On Healing Session.

Remember: Speak them in the present tense and avoid reactive words such as "I am not tense, would, could, should, but, what if, maybe." Use proactive or neutral language such as "I am unlimited possibility. I am free from pain. Relaxation is my natural state."

7. Visualize three times a day for five to ten minutes each time. As you become more consistent in your Creative Visualization practice, you can extend the times.

@ Visualization Technique—Taming the Wandering Mind

Step 1: Find a quiet place where you will not be disturbed.
Step 2: Sit in a straight-backed chair, with both feet flat on the floor and your hands facing palms up and resting on your knees.

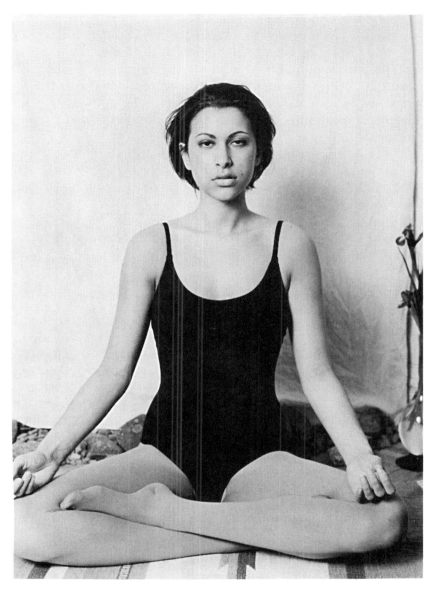

A Sitting Position for Visualization.

Step 3: Close your eyes and inhale and exhale, long and slowly.

Step 4: As you exhale, visualize a pleasant memory or a scene that has a joyful or peaceful feeling to it. A few such images can include an ocean beach with the waves coming into the shore, snowcapped mountains covered with beautiful green pine trees, a waterfall, a large pasture filled with clover and wild flowers, a special memory of a time well spent with family or friends, or a warm fireplace or campfire on a pleasant summer evening. Fill the visual images with bright colors and sound.

Step 5: Finish this visualization by taking a long deep breath, slowly exhaling and gradually opening your eyes. Remain quiet for a few minutes while becoming aware of your surroundings without getting up or moving around.

Step 6: Slowly begin to wiggle your toes and fingers.

Step 7: When you feel acclimated to the surrounding environment you can arise.

@ Visualization Technique—The Vision Quest

Step 1: Find a quiet place where you will not be disturbed.

Step 2: Sit in a straight-backed chair, with both feet flat on the floor and your hands facing palms up and resting on your knees.

Step 3: Close your eyes and inhale and exhale long and slowly.

Step 4: As you exhale visualize the way you would like your life to be. Create a specific image, with an attention to the physical details; i.e., snowcapped mountains covered with beautiful green pine trees, a waterfall, a large pasture filled with clover and wild flowers, the image of yourself in a loving caring romantic relationship or family or friends. Fill the visual images with bright colors and sound, touched with a feeling of joy and celebration.

Step 5: When the visual image you have created seems full and very real, you can finish this visualization by taking a long deep breath, slowly exhaling and gradually opening your eyes. Remain quiet for a few minutes while becoming aware of your surroundings without getting up or moving around.

Step 6: Slowly begin to wiggle your toes and fingers.

Step 7: When you feel acclimated to the surrounding environment, sit up.

Step 8: Repeat this visualization twice per day for 10 minutes each time.

◉ When You Are in Pain, Follow the Following Four Steps:

Step 1: Do a basic relaxing visualization.

Step 2: Focus on you pain and give it a visual form such as fire, needles or a heavy stone pressed on the pained area.

Step 3: Form visual images that will create relief.

Step 4: Remember a time when you were pain free. Create that image for the present.

◉ Visualization Technique—End Your Pain

Step l: Find a quiet place where you will not be disturbed.

Step 2: Sit in a straight-backed chair, with both feet flat on the floor and your hands facing palms up and resting on your knees.

Step 3: Close your eyes. Inhale and exhale long and slowly.

Step 4: As you exhale visualize one of the descriptions listed on the Pain Imagery Chart (p. 136) See yourself actually exhaling out the stress and tension.

Step 5: Finish this visualization by taking a long deep breath, slowly exhaling and gradually opening your eyes. Remain quiet for a few minutes, becoming aware of your surroundings without getting up or moving around.

Step 6: Slowly begin to wiggle your toes and fingers.

Step 7: When you feel acclimated to the surrounding environment you can arise.

◉ Intuition

One of the strongest elements of the Shamanic experience is an expansion of intuitive sensibilities. As you continue to practice inner inquiry and Shamanically inspired activities you will find that you are developing sensitivity to what intuition communicates and you trust these messages more and more. More often than not, this intuitive information doesn't come in verbal or logical form. In fact in the beginning you are not even aware that you are developing this level of intuitive sensitivity.

Intuition may show up for each of us differently but researchers find that it is generally experienced in three specific ways. These are through: 1. physical sensations (kinesthetic); 2. emotions and feelings; 3. symbols and images (mental).

PAIN IMAGERY CHART

**For Dull Pain
Pain Imagery (If It Feels Like)**

**For Relief
Imagine**

Rope tightening around muscle } { Rope loosened, dropping away

Vise pressing on head } { Vise evaporating, fading away

Muscles tightening } { Muscles expanding, loose, limp

**For Throbbing, Stabbing,
Hot Pain Imagery**

**For Relief
Imagine**

Needles prickling on
(pained area) } { Needles shrinking in size
and disappearing

Hot, inflamed pain } { Melting ice pieces cooling the hot
pain

Weights, heavy stones, pressing
on pained area } { Stones fading and falling away

Pressing on muscles } { Muscles becoming limp

Flames in pained area } { Flames extinguished by cool
water

Acid burning
abdominal and chest areas } { Secretions replaced by inhaling
soothing oxygen with each breath

Muscles tight and contracted } { Healing blood flowing in to
warm and release muscle tension

⊚ *Physical Sensations*

Kinesthetic intuitives experience physical sensations that communicate information. They will feel physically "comfortable" or "uncomfortable" about something. This may appear as a gut feeling, a physical pain, or something that excites their heart.

⊚ *Emotional Intuition*

This is usually experienced as a vague or specific feeling that has no explanation, but is usually right. You might feel slightly depressed because you know something is wrong. You actually become sensitive to the emotional states of others who are around you. You see their posture or you automatically have a feeling arise when they say something. It is not intellectual. It happens right there in that moment. Emotional intuitives often say the words "I like" and "I don't like," or "This feels good or bad to me." They respond to requests from others and make decisions based on how they feel. If they are not conscious of this quality they may experience a feeling without realizing that they are picking up thoughts and feelings from another person.

⊚ *Mental Intuition*

Can resemble a thought. It may simply be an internal conversation you are having with yourself about a solution to a problem. It could be a brainstorm in the shower, a hunch, a nagging thought that won't go away in the mind of a person who is not normally obsessive about thoughts. Mental Intuition is not logical but you might initially experience it as if it is. These thoughts are about common sense and what seems obvious. It is a more goal oriented sensibility than the other two forms of intuition.

According to my friend Nancy Rosanoff, a respected writer and speaker on intuition, "Most often people have a combination of the above three, though one form may be dominant. Rarely is someone totally one type. We categorize them only to indicate that there is more than one way to perceive intuitive information."*

*Intuition Workout. A practical guide to discovering and developing your inner knowing, Nancy Rosanoff, Aslan Publishing, Santa Rosa, CA, 1991, pp. 17–18.

@ *Fourteen Transformational Affirmations and Their Related Shaman Massage Techniques*

In the process of applying Hands-On Healing you will be using, individually or in combination, fourteen massage and bodywork techniques. There are also fourteen Shamanic affirmations, one for each Shaman massage technique. Both practitioner and partner should state one of these affirmations as a focusing tool during the session. Repeat it throughout the session.

During the healing session you will want to keep a note pad next to your massage table or mat. As you allow your intuition to roam as you practice each technique, brainstorms and enlivening thoughts will begin to arise in your consciousness. You will begin to have a sense of the unlimited possibilities available to you:

- The fundamental aspects of making proper choices.
- Why you make poor choices.
- How to stop being a victim of circumstances.
- What personal power consists of.
- How to act rather than react.
- The essential steps to preparing a personal plan of action.
- Why people so often fail when they could succeed.
- Why what is rational, possible, sensible, practical, reasonable or probable has nothing to do health and healing.
- The role of self-love in making productive decisions.

@ *Shamanic Affirmations and Associated Shaman Massage Techniques*

1. Affirmation: I deserve love and respect. (Shaman Massage Technique—Energy Sourcing.)

2. Affirmation: My ability to receive love is determined by what I believe I deserve to receive. (Shaman Massage Technique—Muscle Kneading.)

3. Affirmation: If I live with love in my heart I always have enough of what I need. (Shaman Massage Technique—Expanding The Internal Chi.)

4. Affirmation: I am never given more than I can handle. The support is always there either through grace or through the asking. (Shaman Massage Technique—Polarity Similars.)

5. Affirmation: I cannot control anything but through surrender. (Shaman Massage Technique—Chi Balancing.)

6. Affirmation: I am perfectly fine the way I am and there is nothing about me that I have to change. (Shaman Massage Technique—Rhythmic Pressure Point Massage.)

7. Affirmation: Everything in life involves change and transformation. Whether or not I choose transformation, everything is transformed by time. (Shaman Massage Technique—Increasing Joint Motion [Range of Motion].)

8. Affirmation: My desire for habit and comfort is an essential part of the human condition. I will not judge myself for these desires. (Shaman Massage Technique—Pull and Stretch Traction.)

9. Affirmation: Without a vision or a mission, life seems aimless. (Shaman Massage Technique—Circular Pressure Point Massage.)

10. Affirmation: When I experience unconditional love I am fearless. (Shaman Massage Technique—Muscle Hug.)

11. Affirmation: Willpower and discipline without vision or a sense of purpose is struggle. (Shaman Massage Technique—Gravity Rock.)

12. Affirmation: Life is not a series of lessons to be learned. It is a series of messages to be heard. If I hear the message I won't have to learn the lesson. (Shaman Massage Technique—Chakra Balancing.)

13. Affirmation: At the moment I am ready, willing and able to act on a vision, it takes place spontaneously without discipline or willpower. (Shaman Massage Technique—Connective Tissue De-armoring.)

14. Affirmation: The fruition of my vision quest happens at the very moment that preparation and an opportunity meet. (Shaman Massage Technique—Skin Rolling.)

@ Hands-On Healing Affirmations and the Vision Quest: A Clarification

1. I deserve love and respect: In a world of complexity, multiple priorities and confusion, it is often difficult to know what one needs to have. Many people are highly successful, yet they are unhappy. They struggle at a job that is not satisfying and in relationships that do not meet their basic emotional needs. The one defining factor that each of us can use to create joy and abundance in our lives is recognizing that we deserve love and respect. Love and respect can manifest in many forms but on a basic level they mean communicating our needs, doing things which are physically and emotionally healthy, such as exercising regularly, eating well, meditating, getting enough sleep and surrounding ourselves with people who are kind, loving, nurturing and supportive. We must take care of our spiritual needs, whatever they may be—prayer, attending religious services, reading spiritual literature or gathering in community with people who have similar spiritual interests.

Once you have a commitment to creating love and respect in your life, then all of the things that come to one who has made such a commitment begin to manifest spontaneously. More and more, your life is filled with miracles.

2. My ability to receive love is determined by what I believe I deserve to receive: As you go through your normal day there are literally millions of sights and sounds that pass by you but of which you are unaware. Very often we are only able to take in that which we recognize or which catches our attention. If your attention is not focused on having love in your life, then it is not something that you will experience easily, even if it is abundantly available. Therefore, you must not only be ready and willing to experience love, but you have to be able to take love in when offered. If your self-esteem is extremely low and you don't believe that you deserve to have love, then you won't. The choice is yours.

3. If I live with love in my heart I always have enough of what I need: Most people struggle to obtain physical wealth and material goods because it makes them feel loved. There is nothing wrong with great wealth or in having "the good things in life." However, when things are used as a replacement for love, we experience misery. Life is short and death is the great equalizer. The only difference between a poor man and a rich man is their sense of self-worth and ability to love. A person who experiences love will have less of a need to gather material things as a means of feeling fulfilled.

Therefore, if you have love you also have faith and you have hope because, like love, faith and hope are free and unlimited. With love you always have what you need so long as you choose love instead of fear. When you are in a state of fear it is doubtful that you will ever have what you need.

4. I am never given more than I can handle. The support is always there either through grace or through the asking: This is an issue of faith and hope. Living life is the same as being in a school. Your purpose here is to learn lessons, and you are never placed in situations that have lessons in them which are beyond your understanding. To believe that it may be beyond your understanding is to lack faith, lose hope and is the epitome of arrogance. It is only your resistance to reaching out to mentors, coaches, teachers and others who are willing to give you support that cause you to lose faith and lose hope. You always reach your next step either smoothly and voluntarily, or by kicking, screaming and getting dragged. It is the belief that you are never given more than you can handle that creates the experience that you are being dragged. That is the source of your struggle!

5. I cannot control anything except through surrender: We like to believe that we can be in control of things but the fact is, the more attempt at control, the less you can control, and the more out of control you are. Every moment of your life is filled with events, circumstances, variables and acts of God that without support will be beyond your comprehension. Most of the time, you are unaware of these things. Your very existence is the end result of millions and millions of events that have taken place from the beginning of human existence that have brought you to this moment. All manner of chance meetings have brought you to this point. A metaphor given by spiritual teachers about freedom of choice and control is that you are sitting at a table, ready to eat dinner. There is food on the plate; you have the God-given ability to chew; you have arms to move toward the food; hands to hold the fork; the motor function so that you can take the fork, put it into the food, the God-given ability to put the food in your mouth. You have the control of deciding to chew. Everything else is not in your hands.

Alternately control is having a clear sense of your vision and the readiness, willingness and ability to act on that vision. It is as if you are on a surfboard in the ocean, looking at the shore. The wave comes; you cannot control the wave. What you can do is keep your balance on the board and surrender to the wave. This is the distinction between surrender and resignation. If you just drifted in the ocean and let the wave throw you about until you landed on the shore you would probably land on your head and experience pain, discomfort and struggle. This is the result of "resignation." Resignation is not the same as surrender. When you surrender you have the wisdom to control that which you can and leave alone that which you cannot. And, of course, you have the wisdom to know the difference between the two. Fulfilling your vision through a process that is defined as love and respect requires that you surrender to the wave of life; that you learn how to surf on the wave of life like a master surfer; so that the wave brings you smoothly, peacefully and joyously, into the shore to the fulfillment of your vision.

6. I am perfectly fine the way I am and there is nothing about me that I have to change: Many individuals who are committed to the process of personal development proceed on the assumption that self-improvement is the primary agenda. However, this is destructive. If your primary concern is improvement, then you are never satisfied with where you are and who you are. You are always looking to be something that you are not. You are always looking to be better than you were or as good as you once were or you are focusing on what you might be in the future. When people talk about "being here now," when people talk about Zen and the art of "blah blah blah," what they are talking about is total self-acceptance of who you are at this very moment. It means that if you died at this very moment that you would be satisfied with who you are at this very moment. Therefore you do not need to change, think about changing, obsessively focus on changing, compulsively act on changing, or behave in other manners which prevent you from experiencing the joy and wonder of who you are at this very moment.

7. Everything in life involves change and transformation. Whether or not I choose transformation, everything is transformed by time: It is for this reason that there is no benefit in trying to change or thinking about how you will change. If you sat in one spot and did nothing, you would change anyway. From the moment you began reading this sentence to the end of this sentence, you have changed. There is a freedom that comes with the knowledge that everything must change, nothing remains the same. The old becomes the new and it is old before you even realize that it is new. Therefore you can focus on enjoying the process of creating your vision. As you explore who you are and develop your vision, this process will create changes in a way that is loving and empowering without your even thinking about the need to change.

8. My desire for habit and comfort is an essential part of the human condition. I will not judge myself for these desires: When we think about a fish we always associate it with water. Though the water is not the same as the fish it is almost impossible to conceive of a living, healthy, functional fish separate from water. In the same way, there are certain factors that virtually define the human condition. Among these are the need for desire, comfort, habit, relationship, and love. These are not things that even need to be thought about. Virtually every action that human beings take through every conscious or unconscious aspect of their lives, involves the quest for these elements. The person who experiences a state of joy and celebration is one who is at peace with the knowledge that these basic and fundamental qualities are beyond his control. The need for comfort, relationship, desire, and love are the defining factors that all of us must accept in the process of learning to be full human beings.

9. Without a vision or a mission, life seems aimless: When we are young we are satisfied with the physical pleasures. However, there is a point in our maturity when we realize that there is more to the game of life. In many cultures, this realization takes place in what is known as a rite of passage. Though we speak about rites of passage in Western culture, it is seldom that these rites or transformations ever take place. It is for this reason that most people are slaves to the desire for immediate gratification. When people have been through a rite of passage, they transform from childhood into adulthood—not just an adulthood defined by years, but by an emotional and spiritual emergence. At this time, people without a vision or a mission will actively experience tremendous discomfort and aimlessness. It is key that people understand that there is a difference between the content of experience that they wish to have and the form in which it takes place. The content of experience can never be destroyed since it is not a physical thing. It is an internal process that is on a visceral, emotional level. Form can always be destroyed. That is why people with a clear vision may be rich or poor, but are deeply happy with their lives, while people who have wealth or great material possessions but do not have a clear sense of vision or mission can be likened to dogs chasing thier tails. Such people spend all their time worrying about getting more or keeping what they have. Poor people who are attached to material form and have no vision are no better or worse than wealthy people in the same position. There is absolute spiritual, physical and emotional freedom for people who have a clearly defined vision and an honest sense of who they are. The actual discrepancy between the vision and the self-assessment will create the fuel that moves people forward in their lives, moment by moment, minute by minute, hour by hour, day by day, week by week, month by month, year by year.

10 When I experience unconditional love I am fearless: The desire for material things beyond our basic biological needs is an attempt to get love. Therefore, when we feel the only thing that represents love can be taken away from us, we have the fear that we can actually live a life that has no love in it. But love does not require anything material. It does not require getting anything from anybody, owning anything or anybody. It requires nothing but the ability to see God's beauty in another human being, whatever their pain or fear. It does not mean that you are compatible with them in any way, nor that you would even be in relationship with them in any way. They might even seem cruel and inhuman. It is not even for you to forgive them for something they might have done to another person since only that person can forgive them. It is only for you to love them because they are human and because we all deserve love. And so, when you are able to love without conditions, without material ownership, without the insatiable desire for material gain, then you can be fearless because there is nothing that can be taken away from you.

11. Willpower and discipline without vision or a sense of purpose is struggle: When you watch people who are extrmely dedicated to their art or craft, possibly dancers or famous musicians, it may appear that their dedication and discipline is so intense that it is beyond your conception. However, if you talked to these people, they would tell you they are not struggling; they are doing all that they can conceive of. They have a deep sense that to do anything but act on their vision would cause discomfort that is beyond their imagination. They see doing anything other than what they are doing as inconceivable. You may see what they are doing to be so difficult as to be inconceivable. The defining factor between you and them? They have a clear vision. Therefore, it is key that, if people wish to have emotional gratification in their lives and spiritual fulfillment, then they must have a vision. Many people confuse having a vision with having a goal. They are not the same. A vision does not have any particular form. It is a way of being that is loving, respectful, and nurturing to the point that, when the day comes to its end, you know that you have lived life fully. Goals are defined by physical forms and all physical forms can decay or change. People with a vision can have their vision even if they are in solitary confinement. People attached to goals are the same as people attached to material wealth, always struggling for more or afraid of losing what they have. When your vision is clear and you are honest in your self-assessment, then whatever physical events are required to make that vision a reality just happens, poof, as if by magic. Is it magic? No, it's just the way life works.

12. Life is not a series of lessons to be learned. It is a series of messages to be heard. If I hear the message I won't have to learn the lesson: This is a concept that is difficult for many people to understand, because so many theories about success tell us that achievement is the end result of a long uphill battle in a hostile world. The truth is that we are always doing something at every second, and the things that we are most ready, willing and able to do, we do without thought. It is an effortless process. When you are hungry you are ready willing and able to eat. Breathing or awakening from a long sleep are things that simply happen. When it is time for something, it is time and it happens because it can do nothing else but happen. It is important for a person who is committed to a joyous and struggle-free life to take a few moments every morning and explore things and then decide to do those things that will create a desired result and which can be done as easily as taking a deep breath.

13. At the moment I am ready, willing and able to act on a vision, it takes place spontaneously without discipline or willpower: It is easy to see things as good or bad, however, it is really only effective to do this concerning moral issues. When we look back at our lives we can all see times when things that seemed positive later turned out to be the foundation for disasters and other things, which though appearing negative at the time, turned out to be great gifts. It is seldom that we can clearly see the long-term benefits or potential damage inherent in a particular event at a particular time. Therefore, it is important to understand that when your foundation is love and respect, everything that happens in your life is a gift.

14. The fruition of my vision quest happens at the very moment that preparation and an opportunity meet: Experience this by practicing the following simple exercise.

1. Close your eyes and pick a color in your mind.

2. Open your eyes and carefully look around the room for the color you have chosen. Look at the details of the room for the color—pictures, chair legs, trimmings, accessories, etc.

Did you notice these colors in the room before you did this exercise? Probably not. The point is that they were there all the time. But your attention wasn't on them. When you are prepared to see a certain color in the room the opportunity arises immediately. There it is! There all the time. When you are prepared for miracles, they will happen. And they were already happening. You were simply looking in another direction.

◉ Breathing to a Shamanic State

Massage and healing touch is often associated with reducing pain and stress, but touch also has a healing and balancing quality for the emotions and the spirit. There are many different approaches that one can use to open those areas where repressed emotions are stored. The use of intense breathing and sound are among the most effective. When you breathe deeply and exhale forcefully or scream repeatedly, a deep emotional release may take place. This release takes place in convulsive, orgasm-like waves that begin in the pelvis and spread throughout the body. If working with a partner, one can do deep circular rhythmic pressure and skin rolling while the other acts out his or her physical or emotional pain with the face, voice, or body. In time this may trigger the memory and release of early emotional traumas.

As you are breathing deeply and using sound as a release factor it may be very helpful to make unusual faces. Often a set facial expression will be a part of the individual's body armor. For example, someone who smiles when relating tragic events may be blocking his or her true feelings. If you are working with a partner you can have him or her push on your chest while you are making different sounds or screaming.

Many healers and Shamanic practitioners will create different distinctions and domains within the individual to facilitate their work. Some of these, like the division of the body into systems [i.e. muscular system, respiratory, glandular, nervous system, etc.] are accepted among most health care workers. Many bodyworkers divide the body into large segments: head, torso, pelvis, legs, feet and when doing body/mind energy release work or healing believe that when a person experiences major energy blocks, these blocks are located in seven specific segments of the body: around the eyes, the mouth, the neck, the chest (including the arms), the diaphragm, the abdomen, and the pelvis (including the legs). Shamanic practitioners may see the individual through the Chakras and/or the five elements. Thus a health problem or a particular organ, muscle or action may be seen as ether, air, fire, water or earth. Though all of these distinctions are physically connected they are energetically independent. At the same time they each have a strong physical reaction with each other.

Which is the best system to work with? It all depends on where your own interests lie. Whichever approach you use, the fact remains that a reduction of the armoring in one segment may result in increased armoring in another, as a way of compensating. Until a state of wholeness and balance is brought about, compensation will occur. If one energy center contains too much Chi or Prana, some other energy center usually has too little; if a person has an imbalance in the temporomandibular joint, knee or back pain may be the compensation factor. If the emotional blockage is too strong it may cause a weakness in the physical domain and if a person is spiritually distraught this may appear as a mental weakness.

Throughout the growing and healing process there is a constant compensation between the physical, emotional and spiritual. It is this dance between energy and structure, spiritual and emotional, touch and movement that make the Shamanic healing process so exciting, invigorating and fun. Whatever happens on one level of personal existence will reflect on all levels. As you work with your partner you may both feel disoriented, and experience a wide range of emotional shifts. You may also feel as if you are in a dream state even while awake. Things and people will seem different and yet you will feel very focused, grounded a whole new kind of way. This is all part of what I call the Shaman-shift. You are experiencing a new reality.

@ Tapping the Intuitive Reality

A person in an altered state of consciousness is given information on many levels and in many forms. In the early stages, this information is experienced as an intuitive faculty. This intuition enables you to focus on different choices for decision making and focus on the one that is in alignment with your Chi or energetic rhythm.

@ The Inner Voice

For this exercise you will need to think of a decision you have to make and list the alternatives you are considering. It is best to consider no more than four alternatives at a time until you become comfortable with this exercise. Write your specific decision and/ or situations in your journal or on a sheet of paper and number the alternatives. You are now ready to begin—whenever you have about 10 to 15 minutes of quiet time.

Step 1
Relax, sit down and close your eyes.

Step 2
Breath deeply for a few seconds and tune out from the energies of the day.

Step 3
Think of yourself strolling down a a country path. It may be a path that you have pleasant memories of.

Step 4
Notice the surrounding environment. Is it winter, spring, summer or fall? Is it cold or hot? Is this in the day or at night? Are you happy? Are you content? Are you walking fast or slow?

Step 5
As you are strolling, think about your thoughts that run through your mind. Go over them in your mind and think about the choices. Keep on strolling and enjoy what you see.

Step 6
As you are strolling, notice that the path you are strolling on is separating into several different lanes. The main path splits into many other paths, as many paths as you have choices to your decision. As you arrive to the place in the path where it splits, stop.

Step 7
Next to each path notice a directional sign. On each sign is a written description of one of your choices.

Step 8
Number the paths in any way that suits you, and allow these numbers to correspond to the numbers of your choices.

Step 9
Relax, breathe in deeply for a few seconds and breathe out slowly. Take your time before going down one of those paths.

Step 10
Stop and get a true sense of how you are feeling.

Step 11
Where does this path take you. Where will you be going?

Step 12
How do you feel now that you have chosen to walk on this path?

Step 13
Are you feeling relaxed as you begin to go on this path? Is there any resistance? Does it feel comfortable?

Step 14
Venture into this path and take your time.

Step 15
When you are finished, go back to the area where the paths met. Look at the signs for each of the other paths. Venture into another path as you did the first one.

Step 16
Venture on each path and explore it until you finish each one of them.

Step 17
Breathe in deeply for a few seconds and breathe out slowly when you are finished.

Step 18
In a notebook record the events of this process.

Advanced Intuition Exercise: Add a path with no clear choice, an unknown, which represents a choice which has not emerged to you as yet.

@ The Vision Quest and the Creative Process

After food, water and air the creative process is the most basic and primal of all urges. More than sex. In fact the sexual urge is actually an extension, an outgrowth of the creative process. Otto Rank, an early Freudian whose radical concepts on creativity eventually led to his becoming an outcast among orthodox Freudians, "insisted" that each individual is an idiosyncratic being beyond the reach of diagnostic categories, an artist of the self, brimming with will, free to shape his or her own fate.

"Rank linked the neurotic and the artist, claiming that they are similarly driven by intense longing for immortality, a desire to transcend the anxiety of the human condition. But whereas the artist ultimately accepts his solitude, anxiety and mortality through giving his longings expression in an external medium, the neurotic tries to overcome uncertainty and anxiety by perpetually manipulating himself in an effort to make his life perfect and predictable which is an unfinishable, crippling enterprise. Neurotic suffering is artistic creation gone wrong, turned against itself, a kind of negative creation."*

In the Vision Quest there is a transcendence from neurotic suffering to artistic creation. In a sense, Hands-On Healing is the ultimate art form. It allows the artist to create emotional and spiritual integration, physical well-being, enlivening images, movement and healing through the gift of touch.

---

*N.Y. TIMES BOOK REVIEW, (March 24, 1985) p. 3. Review of Acts of Will by James Lieberman. Review by Michael Vincent Miller.

CHAPTER 7

@

DOING A FULL SHAMAN MASSAGE SESSION

You may want to do a full practice session that is not directed to any specific problem. By practicing regularly you will learn how much pressure to give and how long to work with a particular body part. Until you become experienced, begin each movement slowly and gradually, constantly watching your partner's face for reactions. Feel free to ask along the way if you are applying too much, or too little, pressure.

Techniques such as Rhythmic Pressure Point Massage are geared to relaxation and prepare the muscles for deeper pressure; Chi Balancing and Polarity Similars are deeper techniques that effect a more drastic change. The Gravity Rock is also a preparatory movement that helps ready the body for deeper massage. If you simply want to give a good massage to make your partner feel better, gentle Gravity Rocking and working the Inner Chi Points will relax the muscles and remove knots of tension that may cause blockages to your partner's overall energy flow.

When a person is overstimulated or the blood pressure is higher than normal, the body needs to relax. Begin the relaxation process with long and deep aromatic stroking. The penetration should gradually be deepened and the amount of time for each movement should be longer. The aromatic oil will slowly relax the muscle with each stroke. If the body is tired or lacks energy, the opposite applies. In this case, it is best to work shallowly and quickly to effect a tonifying and stimulating transformation for the entire system. These short and quick movements will activate the body's vital Chi and strengthen the energy flow.

Don't feel limited by these various approaches. There may be times when you'll use short, quick movements on one part of the body and long deep techniques on another part of the body during the same session.

I vary the time I use for each movement. The length of my sessions is usually one hour, but I may apply these healing touch techniques for as long as an hour and a half. If you are focusing on a particular part of the body, such as the head to relieve a headache, you could spend about fifteen or twenty minutes on that body part. After you have done several full Shaman massage sessions as outlined in this chapter, you will have a sense of how long each technique should take and be able to adjust the times for your partner's healing or relaxation needs.

Some beginning students believe that the deeper and longer one presses on an acupressure point, the better the result. This is not so. An important general rule is to begin with a light touch and never apply pressure in one spot for longer than five minutes at any one time. Release the pressure and start again. If you apply deep pressure for too long, the body can start to get numb, because the circulation is cut off.

It is important that you use Shaman massage and healing touch techniques on a regular basis. Many people will wait until they get sick before they pay attention to the care of the body and mind. But emotional stress and injuries and illness can be prevented by staying fit and healthy. Keep your body flexible and strong, maintain a strong respiratory system, and emotional and spiritual balance will enable you to resist wear and tear.

The full body Shaman massage techniques integrate the best of acupressure or polarity, which are energy-based systems, and Rolfing and Swedish massage, which are primarily structure-based methods. Shaman massage emphasizes balancing the body's own self-healing energy flow, tonifying the muscles, freeing the emotions, and affecting the body's chemical balance.

◉ A Healing Circle

If three or more people come together for a healing session it is useful to create an integrated resonant energy. It is as if a group of musicians are tuning their instruments so that they become one. The resonating exercise I have described below integrates various Shamanic tools and should be done before the energy healing session. This will draw and focus the healing "Chi." In the Polynesian Islands this force is called *Mana,* meaning the force that cannot be named or described, but is the source of all that exists, and is the spiritual power that pervades the universe. This force is often thought to be more potently concentrated in certain places, objects, foods, animals, and people. In various cultures this force is also known as orenda, Tao, manitou, wakanda, prana, chi, and logos.

One may experience ecstasy while doing a healing circle. Ecstasy literally means "standing outside" oneself and refers to the Shaman's state of consciousness while in trance, during which the Shaman's spirit or soul journeys into the spiritual world or in some way makes contact with the spirits.

Step 1
Have all participants sit in a circle around a lighted candle.

Step 2
In addition to the candle, individual members can create a simple sacred center by placing sacred tools such as prayers, flower remedy drops, crystals or aromatic oils, or burning incense in the center of the circle. The oils, herbs and incense can be burned as a means to psychically purify the healing environment.

Step 3
Each member should bring a tambourine, rattle, drum, or musical instrument.

Step 4
If four or more people are involved in the healing circle, each person should acknowledge the nature spirits and spirit guides from each of the four directions (east, west, north and south). This acknowledgment can take the form of song, dance, a rattle, a drum, or a prayer.

Step 5
A few moments of quiet reflection with deep diaphragmatic breathing should lead into a dialogue of what each person's need is from the healing circle and what they bring to the circle. Occasionally the circle may agree upon a group healing vision or may simply address each member's needs.

@ Expanding the Internal Chi

1. Sit in the seiza posture.

2. Close your eyes and slowly scan your body from head to toe and back to head again.

3. Slowly and methodically focus on each muscle and sense how relaxed or tense it is.

4. As you find each tense muscle, inhale into it and allow it to relax.

5. Now repeat any of the following balancing words over and over as you observe your inhalation and exhalation: Composure (in Chinese, "shou"), Om, Name. Repeating any of these words at each exhalation while sitting in the seiza posture will quiet the mind and relax the body.

@ The Shaman's Touch: Preparing the Healing Breath

Step 1
Find a quiet place where you will not be disturbed.

Step 2
Sit in a straight-backed chair, with both feet flat on the floor and your hands facing palms up and resting on your knees.

Step 3
Close your eyes and inhale and exhale long and slowly into your lower abdomen (not your chest alone).

Step 4
As you inhale, visualize that your bronchial tubes and lungs are slowly expanding. With each cycle of inhalation and exhalation see them opening up wider.

Step 5
"The Power Prayer: Dearest inner voice, filled with love and grace. Please give me all of the following things that I desire _____

_____

_____

_____

Knowing that these desires may not be in my best interests I surrender to that wisdom that will give me spiritual contentment and the ability to share your gift of healing in service with detachment."

Step 6
Finish this healing process by taking a long deep breath, slowly exhaling and gradually opening your eyes. Remain quiet for a few minutes while becoming aware of your surroundings without getting up or moving around.

Step 7
Slowly begin to wiggle your toes and fingers.

Step 8
When you feel acclimated to the surrounding environment you can arise.

THE SESSION

When I practice Shaman massage I like to structure the session so that it lasts about an hour. I do this in one of two ways.

1. I divide the body into four sections: the front right, the front left, the back right and the back left. Each of these sections is given about twelve minutes of attention with a few minutes for the head and the feet.

or

2. I divide the body into four sections: the front top, the front bottom, the back bottom and the back top. Each of these sections is given about fifteen minutes of attention including the head and the feet.

When using approach 2 special attention should be given to the psoas muscle (between the lower back and the upper leg). This muscle is an important link between movement in the upper and lower halves of the body. When the psoas muscle is tight and inflexible it plays an important role in sciatica, lower back pain and scoliosis. The nerve centers (plexuses) of the abdominal and pelvic cavities are embedded in its fascia. Many people who experience sexual dysfunction can trace these health problems to an imbalance of the psoas muscle.

@ *Where the Imbalances Lie*

When applying Shaman massage, it is important to remember that all may not be as it appears to the eye. Structural imbalances can appear on many levels since the muscles and connective tissue of the body exist in many layers. A muscle may be over contracted while the muscle below it may be abnormally flaccid and loose or even atrophied. A soft body with little seeming muscle development may be rigid and hard below the fatty surface. An apparently muscular and developed yoga teacher may seem hard and stiff but might be integrated and flexible.

The body is a magnificent unit that is moved through a complex series of muscular expansions and contractions. When these movements are balanced and integrated they are posturally sound and beautiful to watch. When improperly aligned and out of balance, they appear hardened and awkward.

Begin by closing your eyes and relaxing. This will help you to connect with your partner's mood and flow of vital energy.

@ Head

Preparation: This is the most intuitive and effective technique for relaxing the entire system and creating a bond of trust and sharing between you and your partner. It will bring both of you in touch with your emotional center, slowly release emotional armor, and begin a reciprocal flow of vital life energy between you. Close your eyes and take three full, deep breaths before beginning.

@ Technique 1: Chi Balancing for the Head Cradle

1. Have your partner lie on her back with legs flat and arms straight at sides.

2. While you are standing at the end of the table or mat near your partner's head, gently cradle her head in the palms of your hands, with your fingers gently resting on the base of the skull. Do not massage the area or apply any pressure. The head should rest in your hands as if on a pillow. In a soft relaxing voice tell your partner, "Relax your head completely in my hands."

3. Direct your partner to place his hands on his abdomen and breathe deeply and rhythmically into this area three times, inhaling slowly to the count of nine and exhaling to the count of three. Hold this position for about three minutes.

4. Now guide your partner through this visualization: "visualize the oxygen bringing relaxation into your body and exhale the tension out, feeling your muscles relaxing."

5. Your partner may begin to feel warmth in your hands. When this happens coordinate your breathing so it is in the same inhalation/exhalation pattern as your partner's. Close your eyes and repeat this breathing pattern for two to three minutes. Now remove your hands very slowly. If your partner indicates in any way that she would like to hold this position for a while longer, return your hands. Do not remove your hands too quickly since this may be disquieting to your partner. This contact when done properly produces a sensation of having the entire body cradled and is extremely comforting.

@ Back

Preparation: Have your partner turn over on her stomach. Stand at the left side of the table or if working on a mat sit cross-legged on the left side of the mat. Place a small pillow or a rolled-up towel under your partner's head so that the neck and head are even with the shoulders. This prevents any strain to the neck. The first technique you will be using is Gravity Rock down each side of the spine. This technique will stimulate circulation and provide a sense of well-being to the whole body. As you become experienced you will begin to use this technique to define problem areas in other parts of the body. With greater skill you will feel heat or pulsation

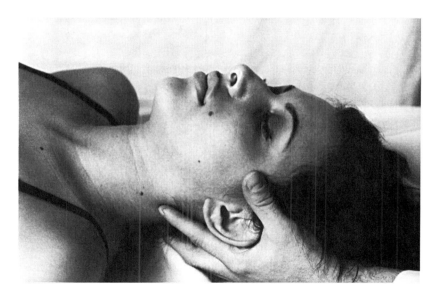

Head Cradle.

whenever your moving hand makes contact with a reflex point to an area of imbalance.

@ Technique 2: Gravity Rock on Back

1. Standing on your partner's left side gently place your left hand at the base of the neck and your lower hand about six inches below it on the left side of the spine. Your hands should be lightly curved, with the fingertips barely resting on each contact point on the back. Now rock nine times using gentle pressure with the palms. Remember to rock gently. Do not press down on the spine.

2. Move the bottom hand about four inches down the back on left side of the spine, keeping the upper hand in the same place. Now gently rock.

3. Continue moving the lower hand down the back in this manner about four inches each time, until you reach the base of your partner's sacrum.

4. Now move your hands back to the starting position, but with your palms resting on the other side of the spine, about two inches away, and repeat the process.

Next apply Rhythmic Pressure Point Massage to the spine with your thumbs.

@ Technique 3: Back

1. Place your hands on your partner's back with the thumbs resting in the spinal groove. The top hand should be at the base of the neck with the bottom hand next to it, as in the Gravity Rock.

2. Make sure to keep the upper thumb in place and move the lower thumb slowly down the back (taking care to stay in the spinal groove), applying firm Rhythmic Pressure down to the end of the spine. Apply pressure six times in each spot, moving the hand about four inches at a time.

3. Move the hands to the other side of the spine, with the thumb in the spinal groove, and, starting at the top, repeat the process. Now apply Rhythmic Pressure with the thumbs in a circular motion on both sides of the spine.

@ Technique 4: Back

Starting at the base of the neck, place one open hand on each side of the spine. Inhale and exhale slowly three times. Move down the spine with both palms, about four inches at a time, applying very light touch all the way to the end of the spine.

@ Technique 5: Connective Tissue De-armoring of the Back

1. Start just below the bottom tip of the shoulder blade (scapula). Grasp the muscle between your thumb and the index finger of your left hand, close to the shoulder blade. Lift and squeeze as firmly as possible. As the flesh slides away, grab and squeeze it with your right hand. Repeat this movement, alternating hands, left to right, left to right and work down to the end of the spine. It may be a little difficult to do this on the lower back due to the tightness of the tissue, but give it a try.

2. Now apply this technique back up to the shoulder blade.

3. Repeat Connective Tissue De-Armoring on the side of back.

@ Buttocks

Preparation: When applying Shaman massage techniques to the buttocks it is important to apply a light tough. This is a very sensitive area, a storage area for fear, anger, and sexual energy. Many people associate the buttocks with sensuous feelings. If your partner is uncomfortable or resistant to massage on this area, move on to another body area. However, most people like it, and find massage on the buttocks to be pleasurable and therapeutic. Shaman Massage

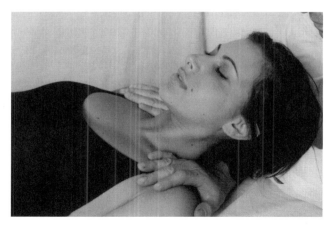

Connective De-Armoring.

on the buttocks is tonifying to these muscles and can relieve pain and spasm in the thighs and lower back.

@ Technique 6: Muscle Hug

1. Place hands, palms open, on each side of the buttocks. Press the buttocks together and hold for the count of five. Repeat three times.

2. Next apply Rhythmic Pressure Point Massage. Place both hands at the superior part (top) of the buttock.

3. Using both thumbs at once, apply pressure and release. Press, Release, press, release. Continue this alternating pressure over the entire buttock for two to three minutes. Repeat on other buttock. On each buttock, start with gentle pressure and gradually increase to firm pressure.

@ Technique 7: Complete the Massage of the Buttocks by Using the Polarity Similars Technique—from Buttocks to Calf

1. Look for a sensitive reflex point by pressing firmly into one calf with your thumb. If this point is not sensitive press around the calf area until a sensitive point is found. Once you have found this sensitive point place your middle finger of this same hand on this point and keep it there.

2. Repeat step one of this Polarity Similars Technique with the other hand. The only difference is once you find a sensitive spot, replace your thumb with your index finger.

3. In general, hold both contacts until you feel a sensation of heat or pulsation.

4. Repeat this process in the same manner on the other side of the body. The Polarity Similars Technique creates a sense of balance and equilibrium in the lower back and legs.

@ Legs

@ Technique 8: Gravity Rock to the Back of the Legs

1. Place one hand just below the buttocks. You will be keeping this hand in a stable, non-moving position. Place the other hand

(the lower, moving one) directly on the back of the knee joint. Now rock your lower hand gently 9 times.

2. Moving the lower hand about 3 inches at a time, move down to the ankle, rocking nine times every 3 inches.

3. Repeat this same sequence on the other leg.

◉ Technique 9: Muscle Kneading to the Back of the Legs

1. Place both hands on back of your partner's thigh (these are the hamstring muscles), immediately below the buttocks. Starting with the lower hand, firmly take a portion of the thigh between the thumb and fingers and knead it moving down the knee. Now knead the calf muscles moving toward the ankle. If you find this technique awkward, imagine you are kneading dough. It is the same motion.

2. Repeat the kneading motion on the other leg.

Note: Do not knead the ankles. Kneading is not effective when applied to bony areas.

◉ Technique 10: Rhythmic Pressure Point Massage to the Back of the Legs

1. Place your hands on your partner's thigh, just below the buttocks. Keep the upper hand stable.

2. With the other, moving hand, apply Pressure Point Massage with palm down to the knee. Apply the pressure by leaning your body weight gently into your palm. Do not apply Rhythmic Pressure behind knee since this may create unnecessary stress to this area.

When doing this, apply Rhythmic Pressure Point Massage from just below knee to the heel of the foot. Do not place pressure to ankle bone.

3. Now repeat this same sequence on the other leg.

◉ Technique 11: The Range of Motion for the Front of the Legs (the Back Knee Bend)

1. Move to the foot of the massage table.

2. Place the palm of one hand on the top of each of your partner's feet.

3. Holding the feet firmly, bend both your partner's legs at the knee and press feet toward buttocks. Stop when you feel resistance.

Remember: Never force a body part beyond its comfortable range of motion. Bending both legs at the same time will help you determine which leg is tighter and more in need of attention. You can then perform more Range of Motion of this leg in order to develop a balance between the two. The goal is eventually to get both heels to be able to lie against the buttocks.

@ Technique 12: Gravity Rock to the Outside of the Legs

1. Move to the side of the table.
2. Cross one of your partner's ankles over the knee of her other leg.
3. Place one hand on the outside of the leg just below the buttocks. Put the other hand directly in the bend of the straight knee. Now rock your hands gently nine times, applying the motion with your palms.
4. Moving the second, lower hand about three inches at a time, and keeping your upper hand stable, proceed down to the ankle, rocking nine times every three inches.
5. Repeat for the other leg.

@ Technique 13: General Rhythmic Pressure to the Outside of the Legs

1. Place both hands on the outside of the thigh just below the buttocks. Keep one hand, the upper one, stable.
2. With the other (moving) hand, apply Rhythmic Pressure Point Massage with your palm, moving down to the knee. Apply the pressure by leaning your body weight gently into your hand. Do not apply Rhythmic Pressure to knee.
3. Apply rhythmic Pressure from just below the knee to the heel of the foot. Do not apply Rhythmic Pressure to ankle.

@ Technique 14: Polarity Similars—Sacrum to Heel

Preparation: Position yourself on the left side of your partner.
1. Using the thumb of your right hand locate a sensitive point

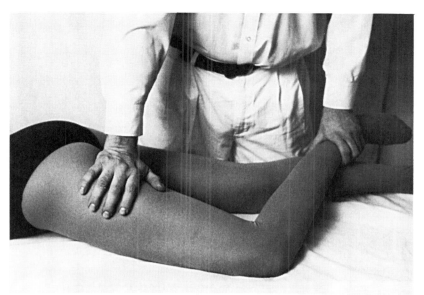

Range of Motion for the Back of the Legs.

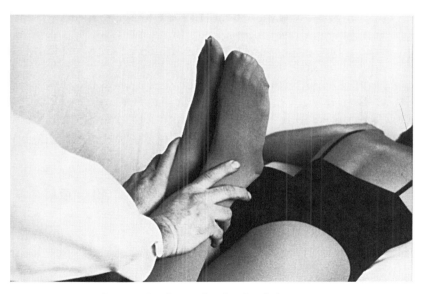

Gravity Rock on the Back of the Legs.

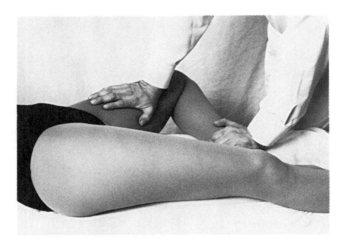

Gravity Rock to the Thigh.

on the heel. Once you have found a sensitive spot, replace your thumb with your middle finger.

2. Now locate your partner's sacrum, by feeling for the top of the pelvic (hip) bone. This will feel like the top corner of a triangle. With your finger, draw an imaginary horizontal line to the spine. This is the point. Now place the index finger of your left hand on this spot.

3. Hold the contacts until you feel heat or pulsation.

4. Walking to the other side (the right side) of your partner, repeat the process on the other leg, but this time switch hands. The left hand and middle finger go on the heel and the right hand and index finger go on the sacrum.

@ Technique 15: Polarity Similars—Buttocks to Shoulder Blade (Scapula)

1. Standing on your partner's right side, use your left thumb to locate a sensitive point on the buttocks. Now replace your thumb with your middle finger.

2. With the thumb of your right hand, locate a sensitive point near the inner border of the shoulder blade. Now replace your thumb with your index finger.

3. Hold these contacts until you feel heat or pulsation.

4. Repeat this process standing on the left side of partner. But this time switch hands. The middle finger of the left hand goes on

the buttock and the right hand and index finger go on the shoulder blade.

@ Technique 16: Polarity Similars—Sacrum to Occipital Bone

1. With the thumb of one hand, locate the sacrum (see Polarity Similars—sacrum to heel, above) and then replace your thumb with your middle finger.

2. With the thumb of our other hand, locate a sensitive point on the occipital bone (the bony ridge where the spine joins the skull). Replace your thumb with your index finger.

3. Hold contacts until you feel heat or pulsation.

Now ask your partner to turn over on her back.

@ Abdomen

Preparation: This is a very pleasant and soothing technique that owners of cats and dogs use on their pets all the time. Every time your pet turns over on her back and looks at you longingly, she's asking for a Gravity Rock. Mothers throughout time have done this to their babies to help put them to sleep.

@ Technique 17: Gravity Rock

1. Standing on the right side of your partner, place your left hand on your partner's forehead. Place your right hand on your partner's abdomen.

2. With the slightest pressure on the palm of you hand, gently rock the abdomen from side to side. Do this for about 30 seconds.

In addition to being very soothing, this technique is useful for releasing trapped gas and balancing abdominal organs.

@ Ankles, Feet and Toes

@ Technique 18: Range of Motion for the Ankles

1. Standing at the feet of your partner, gently hold his right leg just above the ankle with your left hand, clasp his toes in your right hand and firmly rotate 6 times clockwise and 6 times counter-clockwise.

2. Repeat this sequence on the left foot.

◉ Technique 19: Range of Motion for the Toes

1. Stabilize your partner's right foot by clasping the foot with your palm under the sole.
2. Rotate one toe at a time, 3 times clockwise and 3 times counterclockwise.
3. Repeat for the left foot.

◉ Technique 20: Muscle Squeeze to Each Foot

1. Place your left hand under your partner's right heel.
2. Place your right hand around the sole of your partner's right foot at the metatarsal arch, and firmly squeeze the foot.
3. Hold for the count of five. Repeat this squeeze three times.
4. Repeat for the other foot.

◉ Technique 21: Circular Pressure Point Massage to the Foot

1. Hold your partner's left foot with one hand. With the thumb

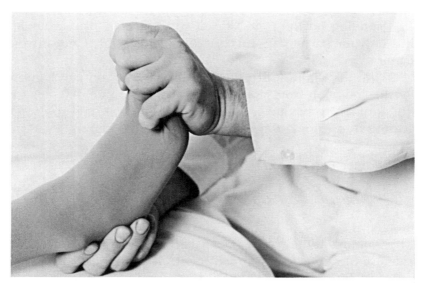

Range of Motion for the Ankles.

of the other hand, perform Circular Pressure on the top and sole of the foot and the toes. Since the bottom of the foot is the storehouse for many reflex points to the body it is important to spend about twice as much time on the sole.

2. Repeat on the right foot.

@ Legs

@ Technique 22: Pull and Stretch Traction

1. Standing at the foot of the table or mat, firmly take one of your partner's feet in each of your hands.

2. Slowly lean your body weight backward, holding the legs as you go and balancing yourself with the resistance of your partner's body weight.

3. When you feel you have reached the point of resistance, hold for 30 seconds and then relax.

4. Repeat this sequence three times.

@ Technique 23: Gravity Rock on the Front of the Legs

1. Move to the right side of the table.

2. Place your left hand at the very top of the thigh. Put your right hand directly on the knee. Now rock your hands gently 9 times.

3. Slide your right hand down toward the feet about 3 inches at a time, proceeding down to the ankle, rocking 9 times every 3 inches.

4. Go to the left side of your partner and repeat for the other leg placing your right hand on the upper thigh and the left hand on the knee.

@ Technique 24: Muscle Kneading on the Front of the Legs

1. Place both palms on top of the right thigh. With one hand, grasp a portion of the thigh between the thumb and four fingers and squeeze in a kneading motion moving toward the knee. Imagine you are kneading dough.

2. Repeat this process on the left leg. When kneading avoid

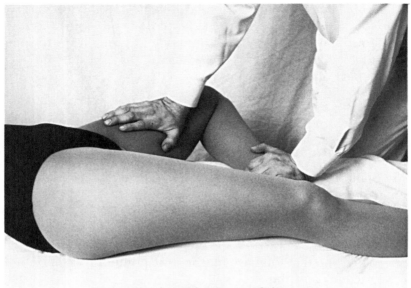

Gravity Rock on the Front of the Legs.

putting pressure on the knee, shin or ankle. These are bony surfaces and do not respond well to kneading.

@ Technique 25: Rhythmic Pressure Point Massage to the Inside of the Legs

1. Gently lift your partner's ankle and cross it over the knee of the other foot.

2. Place both your hands on the top, inside area of this thigh. Keeping the other hand stable.

3. With the lower, moving hand, apply Rhythmic Pressure with the palm, moving down toward the knee. Apply the pressure by leaning your body weight gently into your hand.

Note: Do not apply Pressure on the knee.

4. Apply Rhythmic Pressure to the calf and the heel.

Note: Do not apply Pressure to the ankle.

5. With your thumbs, apply Rhythmic Pressure to the inside of the thigh and calf.

6. Repeat this procedure on the other leg.

@ Roll Your Partner onto the Back

@ Technique 26: The Range of Motion for the Back of the Legs (The Front Knee Bend)

In this Technique, you will be bending both legs at the same time. This will help you determine which leg is tighter and more in need of attention. You can then focus your attention on the tighter leg through Increasing Joint Motion. This will create a balance between the two. Ultimately the goal is to get both knees to lie flat against the chest.

1. Stand at the foot of the table.

2. Place both of your hands under both of your partner's knees and bend the knees toward your partner's chest. Stop when you feel resistance. This Technique determines the tightness in the hamstrings (back thigh tendons).

Note: If you are smaller in size and your partner's legs are heavy to lift, then bend one leg at a time.

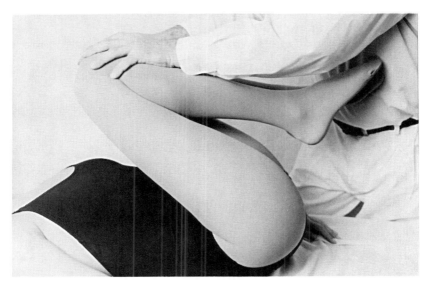

Increasing Joint Motion.

@ Chest

@ Technique 27: Circular Pressure Point Massage

1. Return to the right side of the table.
2. Place thumbs on either side of the breastbone (sternum).
3. Find the soft tissue between the ribs.

Note: This is not the breast tissue but rather the intercostal muscles that lie between the ribs.

4. Apply gently Circular Pressure. Be careful not to apply too much pressure because there are several delicate bones in the chest area.

@ Shoulder and Upper Arms

@ Technique 28: Polarity Similars—Upper Arm to Thigh

1. With the thumb of your left hand, isolate a tender point on your partner's upper right arm.
2. Replace your thumb with your index finger.
3. With the thumb of your right hand, isolate a tender point on your partner's right thigh.
4. Replace your thumb with your middle finger.
5. Maintain these two contacts until you feel a sense of heat or pulsation.
6. Repeat process on the left side of the body side by placing your right hand on your partner's upper arm contact and your left hand on their thigh contact. Use the same fingers on these points.

@ Technique 29: Range of Motion to Each Shoulder

1. With your left hand stabilizing your partner's right shoulder, grasp your partner's fingers with your right hand.
2. Now using your right hand, rotate the entire arm, 6 times clockwise and 6 times counterclockwise.
3. Switch the placement of your hands and repeat this process on the left shoulder, hand and arm.

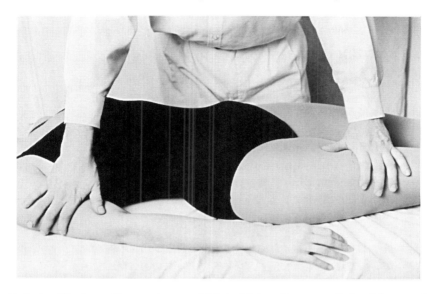

Polarity Similars: Upper Arm to Thigh (Using Pressure Point Massage).

@ Elbows and Wrists

@ Technique 30: Begin with Range of Motion

1. With your left hand holding the middle of your partner's upper right arm, grasp her right wrist and rotate the elbow 6 times clockwise and 6 times counterclockwise.

2. Supporting the middle of his right forearm with your left hand, and clasping his fingers with your right hand, rotate the right wrist 6 times clockwise and 6 times counterclockwise.

3. Switch the placement of your hands and repeat this process on left arm, wrist and elbow.

@ Hands

@ Technique 31: Circular Pressure Point Massage

1. Hold your partner's right hand in both of your hands.

2. With both of your thumbs apply Circular Pressure Point Massage over the entire palm of the hand and the fingers alternating each thumb as pressure is applied.

3. Repeat for the other hand.

@ *Fingers*

@ *Technique 32: Range of Motion on Each Finger*

1. Standing on your partner's right side, rest their right wrist on your left hand.
2. Isolate the finger you are going to be working on by clasping the other fingers in your hand.
3. Starting with the right thumb and working on each finger until you have completed the pinky rotate each finger individually, three times clockwise and three times counterclockwise.
4. Repeat for the other hand.

@ *Technique 33: Range of Motion by Circling the Head and Circular Pressure Point Massage for the Neck*

1. Place one hand on each side of your partner's head.
2. Lightly cup his or her eyes with your palms.
3. Gently turn the head to the right and hold for the count of six.
4. Return to center, then slowly turn to the left and hold for the count of six. Return.
5. Next apply Circular Rhythmic Pressure to the sides of the neck. If your partner indicates that you are working with too firm a touch lighten the pressure.

@ *Technique 34: Muscle Kneading on Each Ear (Auricular Therapy)*

1. Gently grasp each earlobe between your thumbs and index fingers.
2. Slowly rub each earlobe.
3. Move from the lobe to cover the entire outer edge of the ear. This produces an exhilarating feeling and may be done with oil, which will heighten the experience.

◎ Technique 35: Rhythmic Pressure Point Massage to the Eyes

1. Briskly rub the palms of your hands together. This will create a sense of heat and increased circulation.

2. Place your hands over your partner's eyes and very gently apply pressure with the palms.

3. Hold for about thirty seconds.

◎ Technique 36: The Omega Technique

Now it's time to bring your bodywork session full circle. Repeat the Head Cradle (See Technique 1). Then bring it all together using a three-point Vital Force Contact.

1. Place your one index finger in the center of the forehead, between the eyebrow (third eye). Place the other index finger at the crest of the sternum (breastbone), where the collarbones meet. Hold for at least a minute.

2. Move the finger from the forehead and place it gently over the navel. Keep the other finger on the sternum, and hold for a minute.

3. Move the finger over the sternum back to the "third eye." Hold it here for a minute.

4. Create an energetic and vibrational completion lightly moving your hands across your partner's body in a sort of sweeping motion away from the head toward the feet.

5. Create a Shamanic closure with a loving and nurturing thought or statement, such as "have good health," and take a deep breath. This will ground you and your partner, and complete a pleasant experience. I usually close with a prayer such as the following. "I thank the divine force for giving me the opportunity to serve my partner selflessly. If it be the Lord's will, may this session open doors of love and healing for him/her."

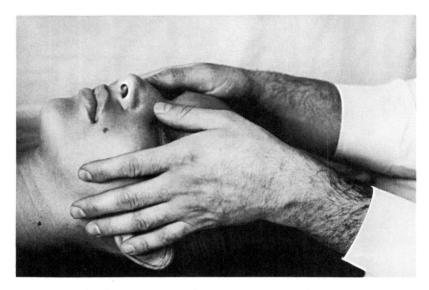

Rhythmic Pressure Point Massage to the Eyes.

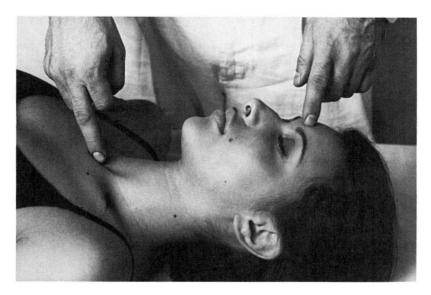

Omega Technique.

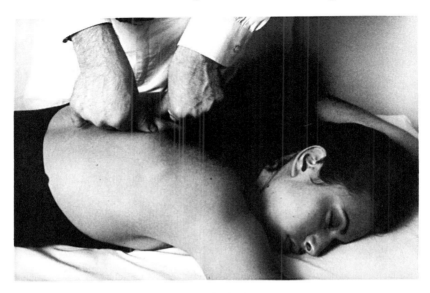

Omega Technique.

CHAPTER 8

@

THE CHAKRAS AND THE FIVE ELEMENTS

We live in a universe made of vibration and energy. The ability to distinguish and sense different energies is a fundamental property of life forms, and every living creature has developed ways to sense various types of energy and benefit from them or protect themselves from them. As human beings have become more externalized in their focus and intellectual faculties have dominated our intuition, Shamanic sensitivities have been dulled. Within our bodies and emotions energy storms occur constantly. This flowing energy comes into our consciousness through what we call Chakras. The Chakras do not exist physically. They are subtle "life fields" vibrating at specific frequencies and dynamically shifting in subtle sounds, shapes, and colors. There are many popular descriptions of the Chakras in New Age literature but the concise descriptions can be found in ancient Yogic and Tantric texts, many written in Sanskrit.

Generally speaking, Chakras or energy wheels serve as the connection between the life force in our physical, emotional and spiritual bodies (Chi) and the unnameable divine energy or Tao that fills the entire universe.

There are seven Chakras. Two, the Crown Chakra at the top of the head and the third eye center (one inch above and in between the two eyes), relate specifically to the Shamanic domain of the inner spirit. The lower five Chakras can be grouped as the subtle energy reflections of the throat, heart, navel, spleen, and sex centers. I work with the sixth Chakra with my own teachers and the five lower Chakras are a key aspect of the Healing Hands Technique and Shamanic Massage. I do not work with the seventh Chakra since my teachers have guided my work in a different direction. Each of the Chakras is symbolized by lotus flowers with differing numbers of petals, which portray the natural division of the inner and outer force of that Chakra. Complex descriptions of Chakras from very diverse cultures using shapes, colors, deities, seed-sounds, numbers of petals, elements and psychological qualities can be found, but in the Shamanic healing work we are doing here it is important to allow the intuition to reveal the details through vision quests and practicing Hands-on Healing. Plants have vibrational qualities that aid in relaxing, balancing and energizing Chakras, in addition to moving emotions. Each plant has something to offer. Realizing the interconnectedness of all things allows one to be harmonious within the physical body of the earth.

@ Understanding Chi

To develop strength against illness, the Southern Chinese focused on the internal parts of the body (nei-chung). Healing was accomplished by specific breathing (Ki or Ch'i meaning breath, air or life's energy) techniques twisting (wringing out) of the body and crouching position (seiza, etc.) for forceful expelling of the illness. This crouching position has much in common with the techniques used in Polarity Therapy. In this position there was a formation of what is called the three outer unions:
1. The shoulders united to the rib cage
2. The elbows united to the knees
3. The hands united to the feet

Within all Shamanic healing there is a process of balancing antagonistic-complementary forces. This would free up Chi. Chi stimulated the activity of all inner organs. When the circulation of Chi is blocked or there is a disturbance of its flow there is illness. In illness Chi may be depleted. We may regain Chi by absorbing external factors such as food, herbal medicine, aromatic oils, oxygen, light, sound, thoughts, vibrations, and transforming these into prana or Chi energy. In China Do-in therapy exercises is to either produce more, circulate, regulate or calm the Chi energy.

@ The Application of Chi in Daily Life

As you develop your inner healing Chi you will begin to recognize that all healing comes out of a balance between the two cycles:

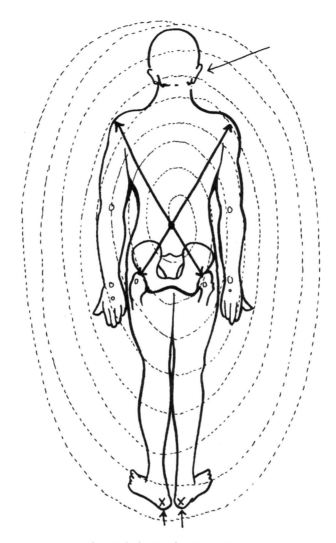

The Subtle Body, Rear View.

motion and *rest*. By alternating between one and then the other in a balanced rhythmic sequence, you can cleanse internal and energetic toxins from the Chi pathways and from the internal organs.

One way of balancing Chi is to sit in in what Japanese healers call the seiza posture. In this position the junction of the toes is at the base of the spine. It is believed by many healers that this configuration enhances and recirculates the flow of Chi energy.

@ Expanding the Internal Chi

1. Sit in the seiza posture.
2. Close your eyes and slowly scan your body from head to toe and back to head again.
3. Slowly and methodically focus on each muscle and sense how relaxed or tense it is.
4. As you find each tense muscle inhale into it and allow it to relax.
5. Now repeat any of the following balancing words over and over as you observe your inhalation and exhalation. Composure (in Chinese, shou), Om, Name. Repeating any of these words at each exhalation while sitting in the seiza posture will quiet the mind and relax the body.

@ The Subtle Body

Some Shamans and people of great psychic sensitivity can see a reflection of this energy around the body. Known as an auric field or "aura" it can reflect physical conditions and emotion states. A "contented" person has a "full" aura and a sad person's aura is colored with negative emotions and is contracted. One need not be able to see auras to be a Shamanic practitioner or a healer. Someone with mental and emotional clarity and intuitive sensitivity can sense the play between these energy centers.

What is most important is that meditation on the Subtle Body will help the flow of energies through the psycho-organism and is a key factor for one to truly advance as a student of Shamanism. In order to balance the "internal life force," Chi must flow freely through the successive Chakras from the Earth Chakra through the water, fire, air and into ether. The all-powerful Subtle Body is a source of strength, intelligence and transcendence, which when consciously evoked, brings balance to the body, emotions and mind. According to Kaula Tantra, "The Subtle Body connects this world with the next. There is no single object or doctrine as important and lasting as the Subtle Body, which provides a constant doorway to Liberation."

The elements are constantly shifting in dominance though we may have a fiery emotional disposition or an earthy quality to how we organize our paper in the office. The elements show up in every domain of our lives and any deficiency or excess in one element

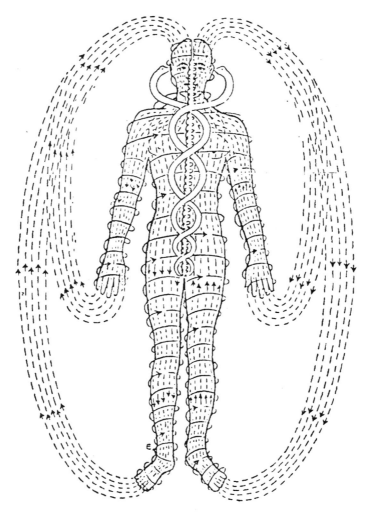

The Chi, Breath and Chakras Merge.

will have an effect in one or more of the other elements. The elements are reflected in all aspects of our lives: astrology, meditation, herbs, the emotions, artistic expression, relationships, color, how we communicate, express love, pray, etc.

Why do the Chakras go out of balance? The Chakras are not static. They are vibrant and active. On a physical level this imbalance is a natural result of the stress of daily living. On an energetic level it is a natural process of how the elements relate to each other. Earth, water, fire and air are like siblings that are always resisting and fighting with each other. Earth can be stubborn, put out fire, and absorb water. Water takes no direction of its own and yet is absorptive of everything around it and can be absorbed by everything around it. Fire can be provocative and can burn if not dealt with carefully. It can evaporate water, chase away air and burn the earth. Air is very difficult to connect to or pin down. It is hard to capture and yet the least bit of heat and it can make a fire even more provocative. After all air feeds fire. Ether is like a mother hen. It is the spiritual link, the mother superior, the chaperone for the elements. It makes them behave, keeps them in balance. In Shaman massage, the Chakra Balancing Technique is a way of stabilizing and integrating the five lower elements. When they are in balance, the higher spiritual centers open and inner vision takes place.

@ Emotional Balance and the Chakras

Within all of our hearts lies a sacred truth. Within each Chakra is a representation of one of these truths. Caroline Myss, a respected teacher of the esoteric arts, explains that the fears and strengths associated with each of the Chakras follow from either honoring, or not honoring, these sacred truths. When a sacred truth is not honored and respected, the result is a blockage of Chi. The result may be physical, emotional, and spiritual imbalance, and trauma and the possibility physical dysfunctions may increase.

Chakra Balancing, when combined with movement reeducation, enables us to maintain physical and emotional flexibility. At times we may develop certain physical patterns which are appropriate for the time and place but are inappropriate and unbalanced at a different time or place. We may respond with fear when we feel threatened. This may result in a hunching up of the shoulders, a clenching of the cheeks, and shallow breathing. Years later, when there is no threat, the person may walk around in a restricted and restrained position in a continuing pattern from that earlier fear. This emotional retention no longer has any relationship to an actual threat and may actually threaten physical health and emotional balance.

As you practice Shaman massage you will often find that certain areas seem tight on most people. Among these common patterns are tight lower back muscles, stiff and rigid hamstring muscles in the back of the legs as well as a shortness along the outside of the legs.

@ *Sexual Healing*

When an individual has difficulty in expressing a balanced sexual response, Shamanic massage will focus rhythmic pressure on specific points on the muscles in the pelvis. The first place to apply pressure is on the adductor muscles. When tight and imbalanced, these muscles can create a strain on the pelvic floor. The limitation in the stretching and contracting of the adductors will actually pull the pelvis far out of balance. The resulting blockage can reduce sexual feeling and the ability to experience full orgasms. By releasing the adductors the pelvic floor will regain its natural tone and fall back into its most effective position.

When looking for a means to release energy blocks tied to childhood emotional trauma and to create a sense of sexual wholeness at the same time, it is the breath that one must address before all else.

@ *The Chakras and the Five Elements*

@ *The Earth Element*

The first Chakra is at the base of the spine and concerns issues of physical survival. In our hectic, materialistic culture, it is easy to get hooked into becoming a workaholic with little time for recreation. Red Raspberry leaf tea opens the psychic space where the vitality of playfulness is key to keeping ourselves balanced and healthy. We go from feeling power that comes from external things to realizing the true power that comes from within.

Earth
In this Chakra resides tribal power. A sense of community.

The Shamanic Message
Love all as if all is the divine.

@ *Water Element*

The second Chakra relates to issues of sexuality and emotions. It is located below the navel. The second chakra is balance, and is relaxed by the herb Wood betony. It stimulates the liver meridian in the Chinese healing system and in my own work has been used to balance the circulation, the lymph and the genitourinary tract. It is cooling for the heat (fire) of anger and other strong matters associated

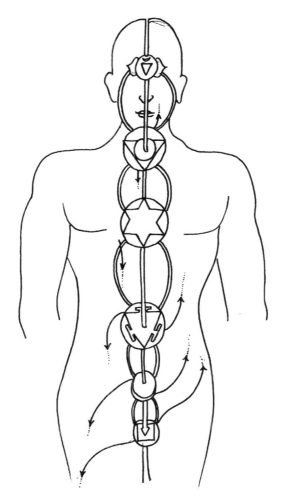

Color in the Chakras (With Crayon or Ink Pen).

with sexual abuse and/or disease. Balancing the water chakra allows the development of greater companionship and intimacy.

Water
In this Chakra resides teamwork, family and partnership.

The Shamanic Message
Honor one another as you would honor yourself.

◉ *The Fire Element*

The third Chakra is located in your solar plexus. It is the center of personal power in your body. Marshmallow root tea softens and relaxes emotional patterns of "control" that manifest when fire is out of balance. Spiritual passion manifests through the fire as does uncontrolled sexual passion. This chakra plays a key role to experiencing divine bliss or earthly disaster. When fire is in alignment there is a balance that opens the door to surrendering to the divine order. This allows for the fulfillment of goals and life potentials.

Fire
In this Chakra resides personal power.

The Shamanic Message
Be true to your own heart so that you may serve others appropriately.

◉ *Air Element*

The fourth Chakra is the central integration point for the upper and lower Chakras. When you are in love, or you are experiencing

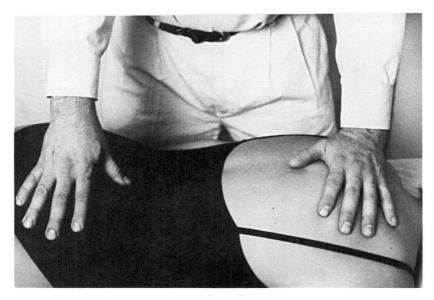

Balancing of the Water Chakra: Where to Place Hands on the Spine.

the loss of love, it is air, the "heart chakra" that is expressing its shift from its previous point of balance. Unconditional love for self and others is key to this chakra and is assisted by drinking Hawthorn berry herbal tea. This can enhance trust in the development of life and encourage one to feel secure being led by their heart. Balancing of the air chakra will support you in getting over personality differences and more in touch with the qualities in relationships.

Air
In this Chakra resides emotional power.

The Shamanic Message
Love is divine power.

® The Ether Element

The fifth Chakra resides in our throat and relates to how we communicate especially to authority figures. This is the domain of speaking truthfully. Red Clover blossom tea allows free-flowing self-expression and communication. Verbal expressions that release deep emotions are assisted by this common herb.

Ether
In this Chakra resides the Power of will.

The Shamanic Message
Surrender Personal will to divine will.

® The Third Eye. The Shaman's Inner Door

The sixth Chakra is the source of our intuition. After initiation by a Shamanic elder or a mystic sage, it is where the deepest level of inner spiritual work takes place. This is the door to angels and spirit guides.

Third Eye
In this Chakra resides the mind soul connection.

The Shamanic Message
Seek your inner truth. Seek the truth of the Shamanic path.

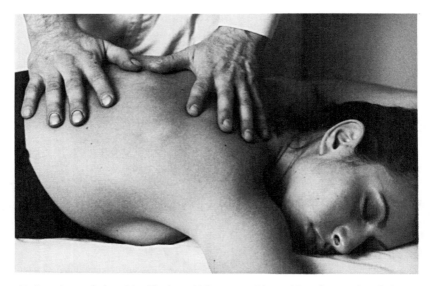

Balancing of the Air Chakra: Where to Place Hands on the Spine.

@ The Seventh Chakra

Crown Chakra (Seventh)
In this Chakra resides pure divine nature (The Eternal Tao).

The Shamanic Message
Be here now. Live in the present moment.

Note: The herbs mentioned in the description of the Chakras can be ingested as tinctures in teas. They can be added to bath water since the skin is highly absorbent.

@ Color and Other Properties of the Five Elements

Colors relate directly to individual Chakras but they also have qualities of various Chakras combined. This simple list will give you some guidelines for integrating color visualization into your Shaman Massage sessions:

Red (earth Chakra): Birth, Beginning, Stability, Heart, Primal Matter, Violent Change

Orange (water Chakra): Power, Glory, Radiant Energy, Sun, the Kiss of Life

Yellow (Fire): Intellect, Joy, Sensation, Brightness

Green (Air): Growth, Youth, Healing, Vegetation

Violet: Transition, Death, Separation, Yearning, Advanced Spirituality

Indigo: Intuition, Seeking, Sorrow, Beauty, Spirituality, Shamanic Vision

HANDS-ON HEALING AND SHAMAN MASSAGE TECHNIQUE

Step 1

◉ *Chakra Balancing*

Place your partner on the abdomen and place yourself at their left side.

Step 2

◉ *Balancing The Earth Chakra*

Rest the back of your right hand on their sacrum, (the triangular shaped bone at the base of the spine) with the fingers pointing up toward their head. This is the Earth Chakra Point.

Step 3

◉ *Balancing The Water Chakra Point*

With the back of your right hand remaining in the position described in Step 2 place your left hand, palm facing down and with the fingers pointing toward your partner's head approximately 3 to 5 inches above the top of the sacrum. This may feel a little awkward on your left wrist. Hold this position as you take three long deep breaths. Now slowly turn your left hand as it rests lightly in the same position on the spine so that it is pointing horizontally. Take 10 long diaphragmatic breaths.

Step 4

◉ *Balancing the Fire Chakra Point*

With your right hand remaining in the position described in Step 2 place your left hand, palm facing down and with the fingers pointing toward your partner's head in the center of the back, midway between the sacrum and the occipital bone (the bone at the back of the head). This may still feel a little awkward on your left wrist though less than it did in Step 3. Hold this position as you take 3 long deep breaths. Now slowly turn your left hand as it rests lightly in the same position on the spine so that it is pointing horizontally. Take 10 long diaphragmatic breaths.

Step 5

◉ *Balancing the Air Chakra Point*

With your right hand remaining in the position described in Step 2, place your left hand between the shoulder blades. As in the previous steps, this should be done with the palm facing down and with the fingers pointing toward your partner's head. Hold this position as you take 3 long deep breaths. Now slowly turn your left hand as it rests lightly in the same position on the spine so that it is pointing horizontally. Take 10 long diaphragmatic breaths.

Step 6

◉ *Balancing the Ether (Essence) Chakra Point*

With your right hand remaining in the position described in Step 2, place your left hand on the point of the spine where the neck meets the top of the shoulders. As in the previous steps, this should be done with the palm facing down and with the fingers pointing toward your partner's head. Hold this position as you take 3 long deep breaths. Now slowly turn your left hand as it rests lightly in the same position on the spine so that it is pointing horizontally. Take 10 long diaphragmatic breaths.

Step 7

◉ *Ether—Earth Chakra Link-Up*

Take the back of your right hand which should be presently resting on the sacrum and turn it over so that it is resting on the sacrum palm down with the fingers pointing up toward their head. Now slowly turn your right hand so that it is pointing horizontally.

Step 8

@ *Integrating Physical and Emotional Factors*

At this time your left palm should be resting horizontally on the neck-shoulder area and your right hand should be resting horizontally on the sacrum. Slowly begin to rock the sacrum area very gently (gravity rock) horizontally while keeping the left hand stationary. Do this for about 2 or 3 minutes with your eyes closed. When you have slowed the rocking to a complete stop, stand with your hands in position while taking long slow deep breaths without moving your hands. Let them rest in position.

Step 9

@ *Completion*

Place a few drops of Sage oil on your hands and rub them vigorously together. Now place your left and right palms at the top of their shoulders. The left hand on the right side and the right hand on the right side. Now slowly slide your hands down from the top of the shoulders to the tips of the toes in a brushing off motion. Repeat this 3 times.

@ *The Shaman's Prayer*

This is a basic prayer I often use at the end of my Chakra Balancing sessions. "May I use my gift to serve my partner without attachment or expectation and may they receive the knowledge, wisdom or healing they require to keep them in divine light."

One of my students shared the following prayer with me. "Through the grace of the divine power and the angels and spirit guides who serve through that power I come unto thee now. Allow me to serve and be myself served through this service. Teach me never to injure, to heal or to give solace, and to ease the way toward your light when appropriate. May I always be aware of your presence and my work as a reflection of your presence. Let me give where it is needed without attachment or expectation. I shall always be grateful to walk in thy Divine Light so long as you may please. AMEN."

CHAPTER 9

@

SHAMANIC
SELF-MASSAGE

Traditionally, practicing any type of massage or bodywork requires that you work with a partner. In Shaman Massage there are a number of techniques that do not require a partner, though most people have no idea how to apply self massage techniques. Self-massage rejuvenates the skin, improves muscle tone and promotes youthfulness.

In the Ayurvedic medicine of India, a technique called abhyanga is recommended. This ten-minute massage is designed to start off each morning in maximum health.

This series of self-massage techniques is easy to master and useful not only to reduce stress and relax you, but for specific problems as well.

Healing is about awareness. The greater your inner awareness, the more you connect to your own body. This connectedness will also help you experience greater awareness when you use healing hands with others. This technique can be applied to reduce your own pain, stress, headaches or backaches.

In my own work I have found that many of my clients were out of touch with their own bodies. Many were not even aware of great tension and stress that they were carrying around with them. I knew that it would be of value for them to develop a self-healing program using touch. As they began to "hear the inner voice" of their own bodies, they learned to apply pressure point massage to tired feet and to send "Healing Energy" within. They experienced a heightened awareness of their sensitivities and imbalances.

These self-healing touch techniques are simple to apply and produce immediate benefit. Some techniques work not only with healing energy but integrate movement and bending to reach some body parts.

In the techniques described in this chapter I have explained the body position required when areas may be difficult to reach.

Note: If you have soreness or pain caused by an injury it is best to go to a healer, physician or massage professional.

@ Polarity Squat

This is one of the most balancing and powerful techniques that you can do. It reduces stress, releases tension, increases sexual energy, and balances posture. It is especially energizing for congested Chi throughout the back and neck. Since imbalances and trauma in the sacrum and associated pelvic girdle is the source for the blockage of healing energy, anything that releases that energy is extremely valuable. By stretching the calf and thigh muscles, the squat brings a greater openness to the pelvic girdle. Women who wear high heels are known to have tight calves and pelvic imbalance. the squat is especially helpful for them and for all people with general back problems. Seiza aids in proper diaphragmatic breathing. This type of breathing pattern is essential to the balancing of contractive and expansive energy forces in the body.

Step 1
Standing, spread your legs about two feet apart with your toes pointed at a 45-degree angle.

Step 2
With your feet flat on the floor, slowly bend into a squatting position. As you do this your heels may begin to lift off. Your entire foot must remain on the floor. If you are unable to get into a squatting position without losing your balance, you may (a) lean back against a wall or (b) place a book under your heels. Remember that your weight should be on your heels and not on your toes.

Step 3
Position your elbows between your knees and clasp your hands behind your head.

Step 4
Slowly pull your head down between your knees. As you do this you should begin to feel a tension or pulling sensation in your upper back.

Step 5
At the point at which the tension begins to feel uncomfortable stop pulling your head down and hold your position for about 30 seconds.

Step 6
If you practice this exercise regularly you will gradually increase the time until you are able to hold the position for 3 to 5 minutes.

@ The Floating Crown (The Head Float)

This technique is effective for reducing stiffness in the shoulders and neck.

Step 1
Sitting in a straight-backed chair, place your feet flat on the floor and rest your back against the back of the chair.

Step 2
Close your eyes and imagine that you have a string attached to the center of the top of your head and there's a balloon floating at the end of it.

Step 3
Keeping your eyes closed, visualize the balloon floating up toward the sky, lifting your head upward off your neck and shoulders. If you do this correctly, you will actually feel your shoulders lowering and relaxing.

@ Scalp Tension Releases I

This self-massage technique will stimulate circulation in your scalp. This will help you reduce tension and headaches while increasing the health of your hair. It is also a valuable technique for revitalization when you are fatigued from some mental effort and you still have more work to do.

Step 1
Apply Circular Pressure Point Massage on your scalp, using all of your fingers. Do not rub or slide the fingers across the scalp; rather,

use your fingers to move and loosen the scalp, rotating the entire hand. Rubbing the fingers back and forth is not only ineffective, but also is damaging to your hair. Do not focus your massage in one spot. Move around the scalp lifting your hands and placing them on different parts of the scalp. Use this technique for about 30 seconds.

Step 2
Grasp a one- or two-inch thick strand of hair between your thumb and index finger, close to the scalp, and gently tug the hair for a few seconds. It should not be painful.

Step 3
Gently tap all ten of your fingers in a "dance" all over your head for about 30 seconds. It should make your scalp feel warm and tingly.

@ The Healing Bridge (Neck, Scalp, Shoulder Tension Release)

Step 1
Pour a tablespoon of sweet almond oil or olive oil onto the scalp.

Step 2
Vigorously massage with the flat of the hand in small, circular strokes, as if shampooing.

Step 3
Next, use gentler strokes to massage the face, ears and temples.

Step 4
Adding more oil when necessary, knead neck and shoulders, then briskly massage the arms, using a circular motion at the shoulder joints and elbows and long strokes on the flat areas.

@ Auricular Reflexology (Forehead and Ear Rub)

This technique, combined with the nose-tension release and the eye-tension release (see below) will relax your facial muscles.

Step 1
Place your palms about one-half inch apart in the center of your forehead.

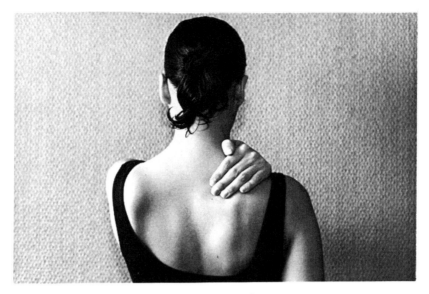

The Healing Bridge.

Step 2
Rub toward the center in large circular motions, applying gentle Rhythmic Pressure Point Massage. Apply this technique 6 times in a clockwise direction and 6 times in a counterclockwise direction.

Step 3
Slowly and gently move your fingers across your face toward your ears.

Step 4
Pull your earlobes down toward your shoulders. as you hold this position, apply a deeper Rhythmic Pressure Massage on the lobes, using your thumb and index finger. Do this for about a minute.

Step 5
Using your thumb and index finger, apply Muscle Kneading to the entire ear.

Note: These ear techniques are valuable in helping to relax the temporomandibular joint (TMJ), at the back of the jaw. Stress and tension in the TMJ is the source of many structural problems including grinding of the teeth while sleeping (bruxism).

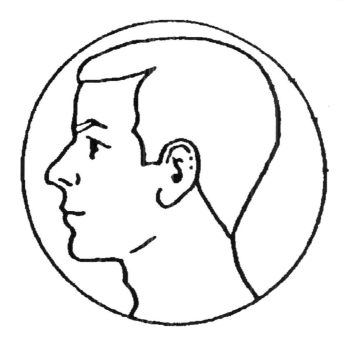

Auricular Therapy (Pressure Point Massage on the Ear).

@ Eye Tension Release

Step 1
Using your thumb, apply firm Rhythmic Pressure Massage along the superior orbital ridge (the bone above the eye, starting at the inner corner). When you make contact with a sensitive point, hold until the pain begins to subside.

Step 2
Briskly rub your palms together until you begin to feel heat or a sense of warmth. With your eyes closed, place your palms over your eyes and apply gentle pressure. Hold them gently there for a count of twelve. This technique is wonderful for relaxing strained eye muscles and reducing eye fatigue.

@ Nose Tension Release

This technique will help to open nasal passages as well as to minimize the vertical aging lines that form from the nose to the corners of the mouth.

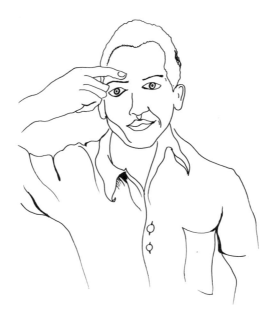

Eye Tension Release over the
Entire Eye.

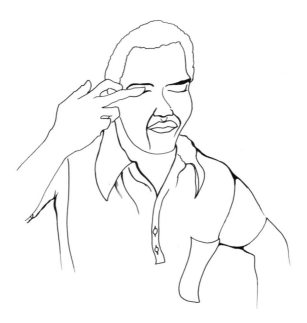

Eye Tension and Headache Release.

Step 1
Place your thumbs into the nostrils and index fingers on the outside of the nose.

Step 2
Firmly but slowly pull the nose in an outward and downward direction and release slowly. Repeat this 15 times.

@ *Temple Tension Release*

Step 1
Place your palms above your temples.

Step 2
As you do Step 1, rest your fingers at the top of your head so that the tips meet.

Step 3
Perform Circular Pressure Point Massage with your palms 12 times.

@ *Forehead Press*

Step 1
Sit at a table or desk. Place one elbow on the table, as though you were going to arm wrestle, but with your palm facing you.

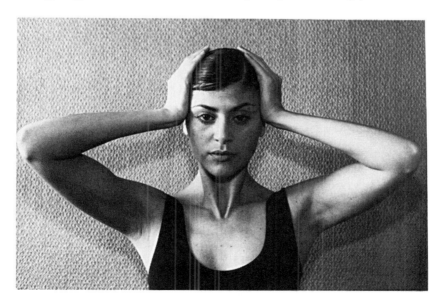

Temple Tension Release.

Step 2
Lay your head in your open palm. Now apply General Rhythmic Pressure to your forehead with your palm. If you want to increase the pressure, lean your head more deeply into your hand. Do this 12 times.

@ *Neck Squeeze*

Step 1
Place your palm over the back of the neck near the shoulders.

Step 2
Stretch your fingers and squeeze the neck.

Step 3
As you squeeze move from the shoulders to the point where the neck meets the head.

Step 4
Do this 4 times.

@ *Balancing The Throat*

This technique relaxes throat muscles and helps to balance the Air Element. It can be used as an aid in the more effective and correct use of the voice by singers and those who speak a lot.

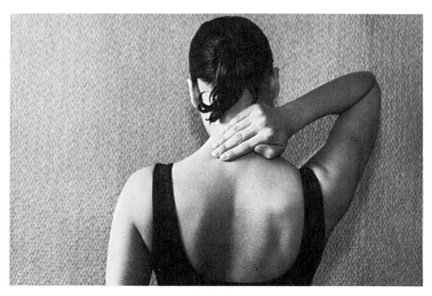

Neck Squeeze.

Step 1

Apply very gentle Rhythmic Pressure Point Massage with your thumb and middle finger along the side of your throat. If the pressure is uncomfortable lighten your touch.

Step 2

Move from the bottom of the throat to the jawbone 4 times.

Step 3

Inhale and exhale deeply through your mouth 3 times.

@ *Shoulder Tension Release*

Step 1

Place either hand across your chest.

Step 2

Grasp the top of the opposite shoulder with your hand.

Step 3

Perform a Muscle Hug on your shoulder.

Step 4

Continue the Muscle Hug as far down your back as you can reach. Continue until you feel the tension leaving the area.

Step 5

Repeat Steps 1 through 4 with your opposite hand on the opposite shoulder. This will release tension in the shoulders and upper back.

Step 6

With your arms in the same position, apply firm Rhythmic Pressure Point Massage with your middle finger from your back up to your ear.

@ *Frontal Arm and Chest Muscle Balancing*

Step 1

With one hand, grab your opposing forearm just above the wrist.

Step 2

Hold the muscle in the web between your thumb and fingers.

Step 3
Squeeze the muscle, moving up to the elbow, over this bone, and up the biceps muscle to the armpit.

Step 4
Repeat 1 through 3 on the other arm.

Step 5
Place your hand on the muscles of your chest.

Step 6
Grip the muscle in the palm of your hand and hold it with your thumb and fingers and then release.

Step 7
Repeat this sequence 3 times and then repeat 1 through 6 on the other side of the chest muscle.

@ *Rhythmic Pressure to Chest*

Step 1
Lie flat on your back and lay your hands flat on your chest muscles.

Step 2
Apply Rhythmic Pressure Point Massage to the chest, using all 5 fingers.

@ *Arm Stretch*

Step 1
Extend both your arms above your head.

Step 2
Stretch them "toward the stars."

Step 3
With your arms raised, stretch each one individually, as though you were swimming in air.

Step 4
Continue this alternating action for 15 minutes.

Note: Be careful not to tense your shoulders while doing this technique.

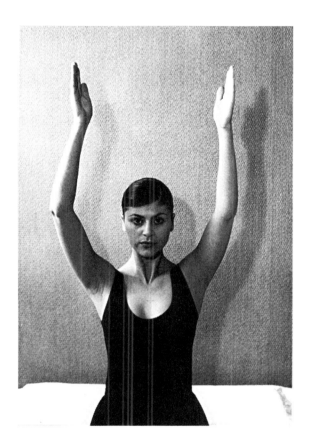

Arm Stretch.

◉ *Arm Hug*

Step 1
Apply Muscle Hug to each arm, from the shoulder to the wrist.

Step 2
Apply Muscle Kneading to entire arm.

Step 3
Repeat Steps 1 and 2 on the other side.

@ *Increasing Joint Motion to Elbow and Wrist*

Step 1
Place your upper arm on your other hand.

Step 2
Pull and extend your forearm twelve times.

Step 3
Grasping your arm just below the wrist, rotate the wrist six times clockwise and counterclockwise.

Step 4
Repeat this range of motion 6 times on the other arm.

@ *Meditative Leg Release*

Step 1
Sit on the floor and close your eyes.

Step 2
Extend your legs in front of you. If you require support, lean your back against a wall.

Step 3
Knead the muscles of your upper thigh from the pelvis to the knee.

Step 4
Knead the calf from the knee to the ankle.

Step 5
Do Muscle Kneading on the inside of the entire leg, from the pelvis to the ankle.

Step 6
Now fold one leg across the other, resting the ankle on the knee.

Step 7
Repeat Steps 1 through 5 the other leg.

@ *Abdominal Balancing (Release)*

Step 1
Lie flat on your back and take three deep breaths into your lower abdomen.

Step 2
Bend your legs at the knees and place your feet flat on the floor.

Step 3
Place your hands, palms down flat on your abdomen.

Step 4
Gently press your finger tips into the abdominal muscles and knead first clockwise and then counterclockwise.

Step 5
Now apply Rhythmic Pressure Point Massage with your palms to the entire abdomen from the bottom of the ribs to the top of the pelvis and side to side.

Note: These techniques will tone the entire abdominal area, vitalize the internal organs, and help eliminate constipation.

@ *Toe Flexion*

Tense all the muscles in your toes. Hold for the count of six. Release. Repeat this 3 times.

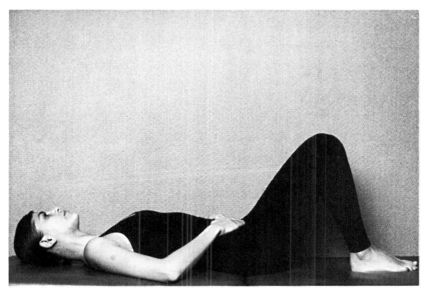

Abdominal Balancing: Body Position.

@ *Foot Balancing*

Step 1
Sit down on the floor and cross one ankle over the opposite knee. If this is uncomfortable, sit on a chair.

Step 2
Gently Muscle Squeeze the feet by grasping the sole of each foot in the palm of your hand and, moving from the heel to the toes, firmly squeezing the foot as you move along.

Step 3
Repeat Steps 1 and 2 on the opposite foot.

Step 4
Apply Rhythmic Pressure Point Massage. This is done by holding one foot in both hands with your ring, index, middle, ring, and pinky fingers on the top of the foot and the thumbs on the sole.

Step 5
With the thumbs, apply firm General Rhythmic Pressure on the entire sole. Repeat Steps 1 through 4 on the other foot.

@ *Creating the Internal Healing Event*

Now that you have developed a healing relationship with each part of your body, you can bring all of these elements together as one.

Step 1
Sit upright in a straight-backed chair.

Step 2
Place your feet flat on the floor and your hands softly on your thighs, with the palms facing down.

Step 3
Slowly close your eyes and relax.

Step 4
Scan your body from head to toe, speaking with each part and giving it permission to relax. If there is resistance or a body part remains tense, breathe into the area and exhale out forcefully.

Step 5
Visualize anything that you associate with calmness, peace and harmony. This may be a waterfall, snowcapped mountains, a tropical shore, a field of colorful sunflowers, a blue sky with gentle clouds.

Step 6
Take each breath evenly and rhythmically from your diaphragm.

Step 7
Rid your mind of thoughts. Experience the energy flowing through your body.

Step 8
Stay in this quiet state until you have an intuitive sense that it is time to move.

Step 9
If your mind wanders, simply bring your attention back to the rhythmic breathing.

CHAPTER 10

@

HANDS-ON HEALING: BANISHING ACHES & PAINS

Do you ever have those days where every muscle in your body feels like it is tied up in knots? You can't move your legs without pain? Your lower back hurts so much, you feel as if you had carried a ton of lead up and down two flights of stairs—by yourself? Maybe your elbows and wrists are stiff with pain? You feel as if you're a hundred years old? Every way you move you feel pain and you ask yourself, "What did I do to deserve this?" Why have you been so afflicted? Why has this plague of pain landed on you? You think hard, but you can't remember having done anything out of the ordinary to cause this agony.

Touch is the first response we have when we need to heal. What do you do when you bang your head? You rub it. Healing touch is a key element to achieving and keeping good health. If you are not being touched, hugged, massaged, you are doing yourself a great disservice.

There is the old biblical saying that as you sow, so shall ye reap. Well if you neglect your essential emotional, spiritual, structural and nutrition needs long enough then you will reap the results. Over the years you may have developed poor health habits that are beginning to talk back to you. When you feel aches, pains, stress, and other types of disease or impairment it is usually the body attempting to tell you that you ignored the message of the past and now it's time to learn the lesson. You've been doing something wrong and it's time to do something right.

This chapter will guide you in detecting specific imbalances, including information on what causes them, and specific techniques for correcting them. Many of these techniques can be performed on yourself. Other techniques may require a partner.

Many of us, before we become aware of the power of our own Chi to heal, often see disease as a purely physiological process to be treated without regard to the person in whom it exists. Although many people have medicine to thank for being alive, the overwhelming successes of medicine do not excuse its limitations. When a person becomes ill, it is not merely a breakdown of the body but a disintegration of that person's experience of life. Discomfort, fear, and confusion predominate. A person can become dependent on others for his or her basic needs. If medical treatment is successful, this only means that the body seems to have been "fixed." The emotional and spiritual upheaval that has taken place may not have been healed at all. As we study alternative approaches to healing, especially those of Native American, African, and Latin American medicine men (also known as Shamans), we learn that there is tremendous healing power in touch through bodywork, massage, acupressure, and herbal oils.

In this chapter you will learn to:

(1) understand the ways that Touch heals, and
(2) to actively engage in the use of Healing Touch, Massage and Shamanic techniques for self-healing and for the healing and/or helping of others in need.

You will be taught to create a healing environment and be given the touching and herbal tools needed to come in contact with what many Shamans call "the light within us that heals." Through learning about and making use of these tools you will discover how your healing abilities can evolve through the simple act of touching.

@ Understanding the Healing of Pain

There are three principles of pain:

1. All pain arises from a lesion (injured or diseased tissue).
2. All healing attempts must reach the lesion.
3. All healing attempts must exert a beneficial effect on the lesion.

Healing with energy is especially effective with pain because it addresses the main source of pain and imbalance; namely the

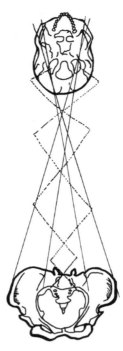

There are reflex points throughout the body. Points in the jaw and in the hips reflex throughout the spine.

distorted vibrational patterns of the organism. People traditionally used heat and general massage to reduce pain but these are not the most effective ways of dealing with tendon or muscle strains.

Traditional scientific and Swedish massage techniques are based on the concept that increased circulation will have a positive effect on a painful area. The goal in treating most injuries is to reduce inflammation and break down adhesions (scar-like tissue that forms in damaged tissue and limits freedom of movement). Though massage and increased circulation can increase removal of toxins and cellular wastes, the fact is that a painful muscle or joint hurts the instant an excessive strain is placed on it. This pain begins long before toxins or cellular wastes would even come into play. The goal is not to remove toxins or wastes but rather to focus on the lesion responsible for their presence. When you address the primary factors that have allowed the lesion to form, you are beginning the healing process in earnest.

The nine basic causes of imbalances in the body are restricted

Chi, lack of exercise, emotional tension, poor nutrition, negative attitude, occupational stress, poor breathing patterns, incorrect posture, and injuries.

@ Concerning Postural Imbalances

Poor postural habits generally come from emotional trauma, from poor standing or sitting positions or sometimes from a particular occupation. Posture is difficult to unlearn. If postural training is not done properly it can cause muscle imbalance and create stress and strain upon joints. Consequently, alleviating pain, stiffness and fatigue on the spine resulting from poor posture must come about from improving the basic principles of body mechanics.

1. When working with long-handled tools such as a mop, vacuum cleaner hose, and garden rake or hoe, tension and fatigue can be avoided by standing sideways to the working area with the feet fairly wide apart and using the tool from side to side.
2. Avoid bending at the waist from a standing position when working with short-handled tools such as a garden trowel. It is best to kneel, using special kneeling devices or the familiar foam pad, when performing such tasks.

@ The Practical Application of Shaman Massage

In order to properly apply the Shaman Massage Technique it is important to understand muscle physiology. The primary function of all muscle is contraction. As muscle tissue contracts it also broadens. Often in inflammation or injury this broadening quality is resisted. This resistance and limitation may result from adhesions that may form between individual muscle fibers with resulting restriction of movement. The goal of Shaman Massage then is twofold:

1. to separate the adhesions between individual muscle fibers, which will then increase muscle mobility.
2. to make sure that the muscle is adequately used after treatment so that full healing will take place and adhesions will not reform.

@ *The Goals of Shaman Massage*

Whether an imbalance or injury is of an acute or chronic nature, the application of massage techniques is essentially the same— namely to:

1. balance the energetic distortion in the vibrational body and the Chakras.
2. prevent the continued adherence of unwanted fibrous tissue.

Many therapists will recommend stretching or hatha Yoga as a means to stretch a muscle. This is not effective and may be counterproductive since the goal is breaking adhesions and scar tissue down and neither of these approaches is appropriate. The fact is, that when you practice stretching exercises, muscle fibers do not separate apart but rather are brought closer together. Rather than stretching a muscle, the most efficient way to break down these adhesions is by forcibly broadening the muscle out. Deep Pressure Point Massage, and the Gravity Rocking and Muscle Knead- ing Techniques are able to broaden the muscle in ways that stretch- ing exercises and movement cannot achieve. After the session is successfully completed, the area of adhesion or lesion will allow full, painless range of motion. To prevent the injury from reoc- curring, your partner should avoid putting great strain or resistance on the injured tissue. The best approach to completion of the healing process is rest of the injured area and continual Joint Motion movement in a non-weight-bearing position.

@ *The Sequence for Applying Shaman Massage Techniques*

There are two primary goals in giving a massage:

1. to work on the right spot
2. to properly apply the manipulation.

This is not as simple as it all sounds, for many structural injuries consist primarily of referred pain. Referred pain is pain that is reflected from a place other than where the pain is actually being felt. Often this pain does not correspond to the point of lesion. It is important on a purely structural level to apply all contacts to the point of actual lesion, not just in an area around the painful spot. Often Circular Pressure Point Massage and Deep Pressure Point Massage may be applied to the site of pain with no beneficial results. It is only an area of referred pain that has received the work, it is not the actual lesion area.

Step 1
Place the entire system (emotional, physical, etc.), especially the injured area, in as relaxed a state as possible. This may be done with The Chi Balancing, Muscle Hug and Polarity Similars Techniques.

Step 2
Apply direct action to the area of injury. This may involve applying The Pressure Point Massage Technique and Increasing Joint Motion to the affected joint. At this time it is best to avoid applying Muscle Kneading or any deep manipulation on the injured area. It is better to massage unaffected muscles or tissue. When contraction of a muscle pulls on a painful scar within itself or on an associated tendon it can aggravate the inflammation.

@ When There Is an Injury

In the majority of injuries the primary goal of healing and massage is to affect the injured tissue first and the circulation second (this may not apply in emotional disorders and infections). Avoid Muscle Kneading or Deep Pressure Point Massage for the stretching that would result is contrindicated.

When working on a ligament tear (minor) the area to be treated may be highly sensitive to pain. Use the Gravity Rock Technique, Light Pressure Point Massage, Polarity Similars. Visualization exercises may be required for 20 or 30 minutes to reduce trauma to the area of injury and the system as a whole.

@ Remember

1. When applying Pressure Point Massage, locate a tender point.
2. Apply contact properly. This means firmly but not so deep as to cause great discomfort.
3. When applying Muscle Kneading to a muscle knot (lesion) always work in a transverse motion (across the muscle).
4. Avoid massaging with deep pressure initially.

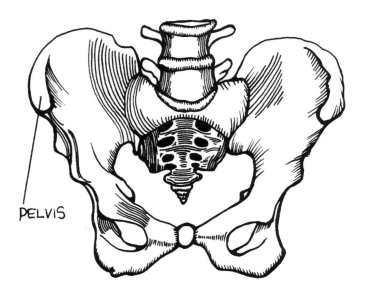

PELViS

Key Pressure Reflex Points Throughout the Body: All Have an Energetic
Connection to the Pelvis.

5. Make sure your partner is in a comfortable and suitable position.

6. Make sure that the muscle is relaxed while the technique is
applyed. This can be done by using warm packs and by using
visualization exercises.

7. After the session, have your partner contract and move the
pained area through natural range of motion as much as possible.
This contraction of joint and muscle should be done in a non-
weight-bearing position.

◉ Healing Trauma with Flower Remedies

Flower remedies are used by many Shamanic practitioners.
Including five of the remedies discovered by Dr. Bach, they are
known for a calming and stabilizing effect in a broad range of
emergency and traumatic situations, including but not limited to
the alleviation of acute stress arising from accidents, bereavement,
hysteria and times of fright. Even minor stresses, such as arguments,
the anxiety of taking exams, making speeches, job interviews, and

other similar situations are reportedly helped with this formula known as Rescue Remedy.

A friend of mine, the renowned holistic dental pioneer Dr. Jerry Mittleman, used to keep a dropper bottle of this formula by each dental chair in his office. He gave the patient a few drops of the remedy before beginning his treatment. He's found that Rescue Remedy helped raise the patient's resistance to stress, while at the same time having a great calming influence.

In addition to liquid concentrate, Rescue Remedy also comes in a cream which is said to be extremely useful in reducing pain and swelling when applied to bruises, bumps, sprains, minor burns, cuts, insect bites, and hemorrhoids. Using the liquid Rescue Remedy orally in conjunction with Rescue Remedy cream is also said to ease emotional upset associated with the aforementioned conditions. Additionally, this cream is also said to be effective in reducing pain when applied to tension headaches, and acute muscle tension and stiffness. Despite its diverse applications, Rescue Remedy is not meant to take the place of emergency medical treatment, but to stabilize emotions such as fear and panic which often accompany these traumatic situations.

When a person is in pain or intense and immediate emotional trauma, Rescue Remedy and Rescue Remedy cream are great tools.

@ Shamanic Massage Benefits the Skeletal System by:

Maintaining posture and balance.
Reducing muscular tension to prevent structural problems.
Improving nutrient flow to the bones.
Promoting elimination of waste.

@ Shamanic Massage Benefits the Muscular System by:

Relaxing muscle spasms and relieving tension.
Improving blood supply to muscles, thus their access to nutrients.
Assisting removal of waste from muscles, especially lactic acid.
Toning flaccid muscles, even partially compensating for inactivity due to illness or injury.
Increasing strength and flexibility of joints.
Preventing or eliminating muscle adhesions from injuries.

◉ *The Healing Touch*

There are many subtle factors that influence how we feel and whether we are healthy or ill, full of vitality or fatigued and depleted. In many aboriginal cultures there is a recognition that there is an internal knowledge, rhythm or life force that influences how we function every moment of every day. They also teach specific techniques for tapping this vital force and maintaining it in a state of balance. Man, along with the rest of the animal and plant worlds, feels, grows, acts and reacts to this internal force.

This life force can influence key aspects of your daily existence. This can include:

- your alertness in the morning or evening
- emotional health
- sexual libido
- breathing patterns
- sleep patterns
- dream quality
- mood stability
- sensory perceptions
- nutrition
- pain tolerance
- healing of damaged tissue
- metabolism and production of hormones
- effectiveness
- memory and learning
- immune health

America has a cornucopia of Shamanic massage techniques. People from Vietnam, China, Brazil, Puerto Rico, India, etc., have brought their traditional massage techniques here and have created a "Massage Stew." Every culture has its own massage and bodywork techniques for reducing pain. There are literally thousands of massage techniques and pressure points by which you can tap into the body's vital healing force. Doing so is your first step to restoring the balance of this healing rhythm to your system.

THE FACE AND CRANIUM

@ Signs of Energy and Structural Imbalance in the Face and Head:

Pain.

Temporomandibular joint (TMJ) dysfunction. This joint is located just in front of the ear at the back of the jaw line. The TMJ shifts each time the jaw opens or closes. Emotional tension and even dental braces can create some degree of imbalance in this area. Symptoms of TMJ imbalance include ringing in the ears, locked jaw, general facial pain, a clicking sound when chewing, headaches over the temples, and difficulty opening and closing the mouth.

Constantly biting the lips, tongue, or inside.

Excessive sensitivity to light or sound.

Constantly raising the eyebrows.

Blinking the eyes very frequently or extremely rarely.

A tight pinched look around the mouth.

Frequent squinting the eyes.

Grinding or clenching the teeth.

@ Causes of Imbalance in the Head and Face:

Air pollution, constant loud noise, excessively bright lights, cigarette smoking, and consumption of alcohol, refined sugar, pork, coffee, or chemical preservatives and food additives.

Poor breathing habits.

Lack of exercise.

Injuries to the head, neck, face, or shoulders.

Poor circulation.

Occupations that require a great deal of mental activity.

Poor posture.

Emotionally based musculoskeletal imbalances.

Negative reactions such as fear, anger, anxiety, and depression.

@ Techniques to Relieve Facial and Cranial Imbalances:

1. Take a one- or two-inch strand of hair between your thumb

and fingers. Hold close to the scalp and pull gently. Repeat over the entire head.

2. Yoga based head stands and shoulder stands.

3. Use a slant board for at least five minutes twice a day. These techniques are good for the entire body and help to raise your overall energy level.

4. Apply Rhythmic Pressure Point Massage along the centerline of the head from the point between the eyebrows back to the base of the skull. Press lightly on each contact for the count of six.

5. Apply Circular Rhythmic Pressure to the neck approximately one inch below the ear. To locate the point, place a hand on each side of the head, fingers pointing toward the shoulders. Slide your hands down until the web between the thumb and index finger rests against the back of the ear. Apply light Circular Rhythmic Pressure with the index finger for about twenty seconds.

6. Lightly and rapidly tap your fingers on your forehead and top of your head as if you were dancing with your fingers or typing.

These techniques will help to improve your memory and increase your mental acumen and will also help to prevent or relieve headaches.

There are various theories on why these Rhythmic Pressure Techniques produce such powerful results. Some physiologists believe that somehow the pressure, even when light, diffuses carbon dioxide, lactic acid and carbon monoxide that builds up in muscle tissue. When these gases accumulate, they may contribute to stagnation of blood. When this happens a person may feel tired, stuffy and stiff.

@ Flower Remedy

When a person experiences feelings of hopelessness and futility, when there is little hope or relief, the physical manifestations of this state may appear in the head and the face. In such cases, the flower remedy Gorse may create a sense of balance and relief.

@ Stiffness

One of the key warning signs for structural imbalances is stiffness. Stiffness in the body is the body speaking to you. It is saying, "I am confined. I have a limitation of movement. Free me!" Stiffness creates and is also a reflection of abnormal pressure on the circulation, lymph nodes and nerves. When the flow of vital fluids is limited, the functioning of the skeletal system and internal organs are also abnormally affected.

◎ To Relieve Pain in Any Part of the Head, Neck or Lower Back:

1. Apply Rhythmic Pressure Point Massage on the back of the head where the neck meets the occipital bone. The Occipital bone is has a strong reflex to the sacrum and thus the lower back. This is based on the concept of Polarity Similars. This technique must be done by a partner.

2. Cradle your partner's head in the palms of your hands, with the tips of the fingers at the base of the skull.

3. Apply General Rhythmic Pressure on the knotty areas where the head and neck meet, using the three middle fingers on each hand.

4. The procedure starts with simultaneously pressing the index finger on each hand.

5. Press down on the points for the count of ten.

6. Move to the middle finger and finally the ring finger.

7. Repeat the process 6 times.

8. When you finish applying Rhythmic Pressure, cradle your partner's head for about 2 or 3 minutes.

9. This will have a very relaxing and soothing effect, which in some cases makes one feel as if the entire body is being cradled.

10. Use Increasing Joint Motion to rotate your partner's head 6 times in each direction.

11. Lower your partner's head and apply Circular Rhythmic Pressure at the back of the head around the base of the skull.

◎ To Relieve Headaches in the Temple Area or on the Sides of the Head:

1. Apply Rhythmic Pressure Point Massage on both sides of your head immediately above the temples.

2. First, hold your head in your hands with the base of the palms placed just above the temples and the tips of the fingers meeting on the centerline of the crown.

3. Apply Rhythmic Pressure Point Massage with your palms; hold the pressure for the count of ten.

4. Repeat 6 times. When you have finished applying Rhythmic

Pressure, continue to hold the head gently in your hands for about 2 or 3 minutes.

◉ *To Relieve Facial Tensions and Relax the Temporomandibular Joint:*

1. Open your jaw as wide as possible.
2. Slowly close it. Repeat this action 6 times.
3. Slowly move your jaw from side to side 6 times from right to left and back.
4. Tense all your facial muscles, squinting your eyes and puckering your lips.
5. Hold as tightly as you can for the count of six and then release and slowly relax.

These are effective exercises to use whenever you feel your facial muscles getting tense. Doing one of these exercises at least four times daily will keep your facial muscles toned and will keep your TMJ relaxed.

Note: Unless it is absolutely necessary, avoid dental braces. Many orthodontic researchers have traced some TMJ problems to dental braces. They recommend that braces be used only when necessary for dental health. If you are planning to use them solely for cosmetic purposes, you should first consult with a dentist who is well trained in TMJ work, cranial manipulation, and the long-term effects of dental braces.

HEADACHES

Headaches can be symptomatic of a wide variety of disturbances. If they are particularly painful, persistent, or frequent, see a physician. Many headaches, however, are a result of tension, stress, or other imbalances that can be corrected with the techniques listed above and other relaxation techniques. To help prevent headaches:

- Use a cleansing diet rich in fresh fruits, vegetables, nuts, seeds, and fermented dairy products (yogurt, buttermilk, etc.).
- Breathe deeply and fully, drinking in plenty of fresh air.

- Develop a regular program of aerobic, strength building and stretching exercises.
- Create a positive environment. See all problems as situations with solutions.

@ When You Feel a Headache Coming on:

- Stop what you are doing.
- Put an ice pack on the central point of the headache.
- Apply Rhythmic Pressure Point Massage at your temples.
- Inhale and exhale 6 times slowly.
- Drink a cup of peppermint tea.
- Sit or lie down in a quiet place and rest your head, close your eyes, and visualize a pleasant scene, such as a field of fresh flowers or a seaside.

THE EYES

Shifts in the energy pathways of the body can affect the eyes as profoundly as structural and biochemical changes can. Among the most common factors that can influence the eyes are liver imbalances, which are often reflected by puffiness, darkness, and bags under the eyes.

There is a theory that information about problems throughout the body can be detected through specific patterns in the iris. This practice is known as iridology. Many healers and Shamans will use this approach to diagnosis. Your eyes are very delicate, and any persistent problem should be checked by a qualified health care professional.

To protect the health of your eyes, make certain that you have sufficient intake of the essential nutrients and breathe diaphragmatically. Eyes need a large oxygen intake in order to function properly.

@ To Relieve Eye Strain and Strengthen Eye Muscles:

@ Technique 1:

1. Sit on a chair with a table in front of you.
2. Place your hands on a table, palms open and facing up.
3. Closing your eyes gently rest your palms over your eyes.

4. Hold for a count of thirty.

5. Keeping your eyes closed, tense and tighten and tense your eye muscles.

6. Stretch your arms over your head, pushing as high as you can toward the sky, and tighten your fists as you do this.

7. Hold for a count of ten.

8. Now slowly relax your eyes and lower your arms.

@ *Technique 2:*

1. Without moving your head, look as far to the left as you can.
2. Return to center.
3. Look as far as you can to the right.
4. Return to center.
5. Now look down to the tip of your nose.
6. Return to center.
7. Look up as high as you can.

THE SINUSES

@ *To Relieve Sinus Pain and Congestion:*

1. Perform a continuous Muscle Hug on the tips of the fingers and toes.

2. Squeeze each for about 30 seconds.

3. Apply Rhythmic Pressure Point Massage to the corner of each nostril.

4. Decrease intake of mucus-producing foods such as cheese, milk, and all junk foods. Get plenty of fresh air and exercise.

5. Use a room humidifier to keep the air moist.

Note: The fingers and toes are rich in reflex points for the sinuses.

THE TEETH

@ *To Relieve Toothache Pain:*

1. Gently press around the jaw for tender points.

2. Apply Rhythmic Pressure Point Massage to the entire jaw holding each point for about 15 seconds.

3. Apply Chi Balancing to the points on either side of the ear. These techniques will help provide temporary relief until you can see a dentist.

THE THROAT AND NECK

@ *Signs of Imbalance in the Neck and Throat:*

Chronic sore throat.
Stiffness in the neck.
Headaches.
Exaggerated tilt of the neck to one side (Torticollis).
Chronic hoarseness, high-pitched voice, inability to project the voice, grinding the teeth (bruxism).
One shoulder higher than the other.
Difficulty in breathing.
Chronic coughing or tics in the throat.
Inability to touch chest with chin.
Bulging veins in the neck.

@ *Your Voice Is a Mirror of Who You Are*

Your voice is a delicate yet powerful instrument that you use constantly. Your emotions are always in action and in flux whether you are conscious of it or not. The integration of these two truths brings us the knowledge that your voice is a mirror of your emotional state. The loudness, softness, pitch, tone, timbre, and expression affects your sound-producing organs which, like all organs, are fed and feed into Chi energy pathways. These pathways influence how emotional experiences are stored and released from the structural centers of the body especially the fascia.

In the Shamanic realm, the way a voice is used greatly defines the response that others have toward the Shamanic messenger. Moshe Feldenkrais, the great movement educator, often spoke of the impact your voice has on others, especially in the initial encounter.

People unconsciously bond to you or distance from the pitch and modulation of your voice. As people listen to what you have to say, they accept or reject or remain neutral. A well-pitched and modulated voice creates a sense of authority, control and self-assurance.

When you continually hold back strong emotions and thoughts out of fear, need for approval, childhood trauma or poor expression skills, chest muscles and throat muscles become constricted and tight. Words can get metaphorically "stuck in one's throat." Throat strain can also arise in those who talk excessively, speaking before they think. The result is pain and chronic hoarseness.

@ Causes of Imbalance in the Neck and Throat:

Chronic tension in throat and neck muscles caused by poor speaking or vocal habits.

Dentistry, modeling, typing, writing and other occupations that require the neck to be held in one position for extended periods of time.

Smoking.

Shock to the neck such as whiplash and other injuries.

Inhibitions in saying what you think and feel.

Chronic, emotionally based pain in the neck.

Poor posture.

Congenital contraction in neck or upper back muscles.

Carrying a heavy bag or pocketbook on one shoulder constantly.

General tension in upper back.

Overweight.

Poorly fitted or high-heeled shoes.

Eating mucus-producing foods that coat and block the throat, limiting vocal range and endurance. Different foods produce mucus in different people, but more often than not dairy products, wheat, and meat are the biggest culprits.

Incorrect sleeping habits such as sleeping on your stomach, sleeping with arms or hands under your neck or head, sleeping on a mattress that is too soft.

@ Techniques for Relieving Chi Imbalances in the Neck and Throat: To Relax Throat and Neck Muscles and Release Blockages:

1. Use gentle Chi Balancing on the back of the neck and over the throat.

2. Use Increasing Joint Motion to rotate neck and head 6 turns in a clockwise direction and 6 times counterclockwise.

3. Hum the sound "ooooommmmmm," projecting this sound deeply into your throat. Then make the sound "eeeeeaaaaaa" deeply in your throat. Repeat the sequence 3 times. Alternating one sound for 3 repetitions and then the other for 3 repetitions. As you alternate between both sounds you should feel vibrations deep in your throat. This technique will help to renew and strengthen the voice and throat.

4. Use a warm-water compress on your throat to relax tight muscles.

@ Healing Movement for the Throat

The hatha Yoga asana (movement) known as the lion pose brings healing and balancing both in toning and relaxing muscles of the throat. To assume the lion posture open your mouth as wide as possible, tense all your facial muscles, and stick your tongue out as far as possible. Hold for the count of six.

@ How to Reduce Pain, Inflammation, and Congestion from a Sore Throat and Increase Circulation to the Area:

1. Using penetrating oils on the throat and on the chest area can be very helpful. Some that are effective are Olbas, Tiger Balm, or peppermint, which are available in health food stores. It is best to place a small amount of oil on a moist, lukewarm cloth. Wrap the cloth around the throat as you would a compress. Leave it on overnight. **Caution: Do not apply over open sores, abrasions, or cuts. This can be very painful and irritating.**

2. Add 1 teaspoon of sea salt to 6 ounces of water. Gargle with this warm salt-water solution.

3. If you use your voice often to sing or speak, especially if you do either of these professionally for an extended period and experience soreness, use a mixture of honey, warm water, and lemon before and after. Also, be certain to protect your throat with a scarf or collar during winter months. **Caution: If a sore throat persists, obtain professional medical advice. Sore throats can be connected with and lead to serious complications.**

THE SHOULDERS

◉ *Signs of Imbalance in the Shoulders:*

Discomfort in the hip joint.
One shoulder higher than the other.
Chest pushed out or forward.
Hunched over or rounded shoulders.

◉ *Causes of Imbalance in the Shoulders:*

Prolonged tension in the upper back.

Emotional stress or high pressure work. Chronic self-doubt and confusion are indicated by tension in the shoulders, often shown by hunched, raised shoulders.

Occupations such as typing, modeling, and certain types of assembly-line work that require the shoulders to be held in one position for extended periods of time.

Constantly carrying a heavy bag or pocketbook on one shoulder.

Poor posture.

A trauma or shock to the neck, such as whiplash or other injuries.

Trauma and accidents that cause a violent contraction of shoulder muscles.

Poor working environment and inappropriate furniture in the work environment. This may include worktables and desks that are too high. This will cause you to raise your shoulders, bringing tightness and pain. To determine proper table height, bend your elbows when you are in a sitting position. The table should be even with your elbows.

Shallow breathing. Shoulder tension will be released more easily as you learn to breathe from your diaphragm.

Obesity. This causes postural shifts as the body attempts to compensate posturally for the added weight.

◉ *Techniques to Release Chi, and Emotional Factors and Holding Patterns Reflected in the Shoulders and Upper Back and to Assist Breathing and Digestion:*

1. To relax the muscles and prepare them for bodywork, have your partner take three long deep breaths diaphragmatically.

2. Use Circular Rhythmic Pressure Point Massage around the medial (inside) border of both shoulder blades.

3. Apply a small amount of penetrating oil (Olbas, Tiger Balm, peppermint) directly on the shoulder area and massage gently into skin. Place a moist, warm compress on the area for about 20 minutes; do not make it too hot.

4. Perform the Gravity Rock technique on the shoulders and upper back while your partner is lying on his stomach.

@ To Improve Circulation, Stretch and Tonify the Muscles Near the Shoulders:

1. Use Muscle Kneading on shoulders.

2. Apply Polarity Similars Contacts on the shoulder blades and buttocks, using massage techniques described in the chapter titled "Doing a Full Shaman Massage Session."

THE ARMS AND HANDS

@ Signs of Imbalance in the Arms and Hands:

Swollen fingers.
Constant knuckle cracking.
Constant finger twitching.
Abnormally sweaty hands.
Constant folding of arms across the chest.
Rounded shoulders.
Difficulty or inability to make grasping motions with fingers.
Chest pushed forward.
Difficulty or pain in the hand when trying to grip something.
Poor circulation in hands and/or arms. This is indicated by an abnormal cool or cold sensation.

@ Causes of Chi Blockages in the Arms and Hands:

Trauma, such as surgery, or a blow to the arm or hands.
Falling on outstretched hands. This can cause a fracture or dislocation of the wrist or elbow (one of the most common injuries among roller bladers or ice skaters).

Rheumatoid arthritis can result in severe limitation of elbow motion.

Irritate the bursas (closed, fluid-filled sacs usually found between tendons and bones in areas subject to friction such as shoulders and elbows). This is most often caused by improper gripping of a tool, golf club or tennis racket.

Arthritis. Osteoarthritis may limit the range of motion and cause stiffness and inflammation in muscles and joints.

Sewing, fine jewelry work, electronics, typing and other jobs that require precision work with the hands.

Excessive and improper strain on the wrist joint. This is commonly experienced by weight lifters who attempt to do certain curls improperly.

Hyperextension of the elbow. This is most common in gymnasts and weight lifters.

Note: When you are applying Shaman Massage techniques, you soon become aware of the Polarity Similars pattern. That is to say that people who have problems in their ankles often have problems in their wrists as well. Likewise problems in knees are often reflected in elbows; and problems in fingers are often reflected in toes.

@ *Techniques for Relieving Arm and Hand Imbalances:*

When working with peripheral joints (Joints of the arms, legs, hands and feet), deep manipulation should initially not be applied when a lesion (trauma) is active. You can recognize if it is active when it is painful even when there is no movement, as in lying still at night. There will usually also be pain to the affected joint when it is placed in a position where it must bear weight although there is no movement of that joint.

Never force a bending movement on a stiff elbow, especially directly after the time of injury or trauma. Attempting to stretch out the joint during massage will reduce rather than increase the range of motion. Inappropriate manipulation of the elbow joint can result in a painful condition called "myositis ossificans of the brachialis muscle." In tennis elbow, Range of Motion is appropriate once the swelling is reduced.

To correct general imbalances and increase movement in the wrist, hands, and fingers, use firm Rhythmic Pressure Point Massage and Muscle Kneading on the muscles of the lower arm.

To correct general imbalances in the wrist after surgery, use Muscle Kneading, not only on the wrist, but on the entire arm.

To correct general imbalances in the arm and hands use Muscle Kneading on the neck on the same side of the body as where the pain is.

Reduce muscle aches and cramps in the hands by applying Muscle Kneading on the forearm, palm of hand, and each finger.

@ *Water Balancing Techniques for the Arms and Hands:*

1. Increase circulation to hands through water balancing. This increases the flow of nutrients to damaged tissue while removing cellular waste.

2. To use water to normalize a Chi imbalance in the hands, alternate hot and cold hand soaks.

3. Prepare two pans of water, one approximately 106 degrees, the other approximately 40 degrees.

4. Place hands first in the hot water for about 2 minutes.

5. Then place them in the cold water for about 15 seconds.

6. Repeat process 3 times.

Remember: Always begin with hot water and finish with cold. **Caution: Do not use hot water when there is inflammation.**

@ *Tennis Elbow*

Correcting tennis elbow requires strength-building movement, while increasing flexibility, and endurance in your forearm, shoulder and inflamed elbow.

Apply an ice pack to the elbow, 10 minutes on and 5 minutes off.

Gently use a soft approach to increasing joint motion technique by gently rotating your wrist 12 times clockwise and 12 times counterclockwise.

@ *Try These Other Three Motion Exercises:*

1. Place your wrist on a table about 2 inches in from the edge, palm facing down. Now raise your hand up and down, using the greatest range of motion.

2. A similar movement is to place your wrist on the table, palm up, and repeat the up-and-down movement.

Do each of these movements 3 times daily, performing 25 lifts each time. By increasing the range of motion you will help correct the elbow problem by developing the supporting muscles in the forearm.

@ *Pressure Point Massage to Heal the Elbow:*

Apply Rhythmic Pressure Point Massage to all of the soft tissue surrounding the elbow for about 3 minutes several times a day.

To relieve arthritic conditions:

1. Increase the application of the Joint Motion Technique on finger joints, wrists, and elbows.

2. Apply Rhythmic Pressure Point Massage to the area around the problem joints.

THE CHEST

@ *Signs of a Chi Imbalance in the Chest Area:*

A structural imbalance in placement of the ribs. For example one side protruding more than the other.

Mouth breathing and general shallow breathing from the chest rather than breathing from the diaphragm.

Chest pains.

Lumps in the breast.

Upper back pain.

Heart palpitations.

Respiratory discomfort and specific problems especially asthma, bronchitis, and emphysema.

Protruding chest.

Mucus buildup.

@ *Causes of Imbalance in the Chest:*

Hyper-expanded lungs that may enlarge and cause problems in the chest area. This is most common in long distance runners.

Poor athletic training and techniques.

Smoking.

Air pollution.

Shallow breathing and breathing through the mouth.

Rib Strain. This is a common condition among young dancers,

wrestlers and gymnasts. In this condition, the athlete places the hips in one position while twisting the upper torso in the opposite direction.

◉ Techniques for Relieving Chest Imbalances:

To relax muscles in chest area and improve respiration (especially beneficial for people with asthma and other respiratory problems):

Step 1
Use firm General Rhythmic Pressure on a line one inch below the collarbone, directly above the nipple.

Step 2
Perform Gravity Rock on entire chest area.

Step 3
Practice diaphragmatic breathing, get plenty of fresh air, sleep lying on your back rather than on your stomach, and use a room humidifier to reduce buildup of mucus in the chest.

To improve breathing, practice correct breathing techniques.

To relax the trapezius, latissimus dorsi, and other upper back muscles, apply Gravity Rocking and Pressure Point Massage.

To balance the rib cage use Rhythmic Pressure Massage between ribs. Move from the breastbone toward the sides. Massage the area firmly but not too deeply.

THE BACK

When a person gets older, one of the greatest storage places for emotional trauma and structural blockages is the back. If you press on the muscles about a half inch on either side of the spinal vertebrae you can feel the hardness and stiffness of the muscles running down the back form the neck to the sacrum near the base of the spinal column. Feel the long hard strands of atrophied muscle and connective tissue. When you breathe, this tissue limits the natural expansion that needs to take place with the breath. The back lets us know, through acute pain, that this imbalance has gone too far.

@ *The Spinal Column*

The spine has the largest collection of joints of any specific bony structure in the body and yet it is strongly anchored in the dorsal area by the ribs and thus has very specific and limited movements defined by the attaching structures.

When there is back pain, massage on associated muscle groups such as the hamstrings, the abdominal muscles or the gluteal muscles can effect pain reduction and freedom of movement.

@ *Disk Problems and Causes*

Pressure on any of the spinal nerve roots can produce pain which may radiate along the nerve and be felt in another part of the body. Pressure can occur for various reasons, one of the most common being a herniated vertebral disk, sometimes incorrectly called a "slipped disk." It is frequently due to faulty lifting procedures. Lifting involves bending the hips and knees and keeping the back straight, which is essential to any stooping and lifting movement. Bending from the waist puts great stress in the area of the L-4 and L-5 Lumbar vertebrae and Sacral areas. There are many muscles directly involved with the movement of the lower back region. All of the abdominal muscles are extremely important in supporting the entire area. If extreme pressure from heavy lifting is placed on this area, great pressure may be placed on the disks and possibly cause them to rupture.

The lower back muscles are small and are mainly used in maintaining good posture. It is the strong hip and thigh muscles that should be used for all heavy lifting work. It is also in the pulling and pushing movements that the strong muscles of the legs supplement the action of the arms and lean the body in the direction of the object to be moved. Whenever possible, try to pull or push squarely in the direction in which the object is expected to move.

Sometimes "Trigger points" are the source of referred pain. Lower back pain may be caused by neural or energetic blockages elsewhere in the body. Occasionally, referred pain from the spine may also cause pain or reflex to points in the spine. This pain is of a less severe nature and may be relieved by various treatments to the body parts involved and gentle massage to the point itself.

Step 1
If a back muscle (this applies to all muscles in body) is very painful or knotted, do not work directly on it. Rather it is more effective to press a point above and another point below (running diagonally) across the pained area.

Step 2
In pained backs, place the right palm directly on the pained area. Place the left hand directly on the opposite side of the spine. This is only for temporary relief. Press on main circuits (the nearest point above and below the pained area).

Note: When pressing points to relieve back pain, begin with gentle pressure around the center of the pain. Slowly work outward to the surrounding muscles and increase the pressure as you do so.

@ *Polarity Similars for Lower Back Problems*

Lower Back Specifics:
1. Ischium to mastoid part of temporal bone
2. Pubic Bone to Parietal bones
3. Symphasis Pubis to jaw
4. Sacrum to Occiput
5. Coccyx to Sphenoid

@ *Technique for Relieving Back Pain:*

1. Lay person on stomach.
2. With person on stomach find the part of the back that is symmetrically higher.
3. On the higher side place ten fingers (right hand below/left hand above and point the fingers toward the feet.
This technique is called "draining the pain," since by pointing the fingers in this direction, I am freeing up blocked energy.

@ *Signs of Imbalance in the Back:*

Walking on the outer or inner edge of the foot.
Back pain.
Tightness in chest.
Hunched or rolled shoulders.
Abdominal Pain.

Abnormal lateral curvature (scoliosis), posterior curvature in the upper back (kyphosis) and or lower back (lordosis).

Tight leg or hamstring muscles.

A stiff neck or a neck that is tilted to one side.

@ Causes of Imbalance in the Back:

Disk problems. If pain in the lower back is fairly constant, has existed for some time, and is very sharp it may be the result of a disintegration of the disk or a rupture.

When desks and worktables are too high, your shoulders will elevate abnormally, bringing tightness and pain. Bend your elbows when you are in a sitting position to determine proper table height. The table should be even with your elbows.

(Do not self-treat a condition like this. See a therapist skilled with experience working on disk problems, such as an orthopedist, chiropractor, osteopath, Feldenkrais Movement practitioner or Alexander Technique practitioner.)

Working in a sitting position for extended periods. This can tighten calf muscles and hamstrings and cause severe chronic backache.

Poor dance or athletic training.

Infection or malfunction of any internal organs such as the kidney, liver, or pancreas.

Infections in the spinal structure, especially in the disk spaces.

Dislocations or fractures, especially to the vertebrae.

Poor posture, especially when lifting heavy objects.

Bone diseases, including osteoporosis (often caused by the use of corticosteroid drugs used to treat arthritis) and osteomalacia (softening of the bones caused by vitamin D deficiency in an adult).

Imbalances in other body parts and organs, especially the abdomen, ovaries, uterus, prostate gland, and fallopian tubes.

Wearing high heels.

Abnormal curvature of the spine (kyphosis, lordosis, scoliosis).

@ Techniques for Relieving Back Imbalances:

1. Use diaphragmatic breathing exercises to strengthen the abdominal muscles.

2. Reduce stress on the back by strengthening the gluteal muscles (buttocks).

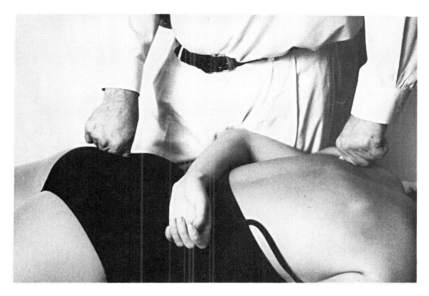

Polarity Similars: Buttocks to Shoulder Blade.

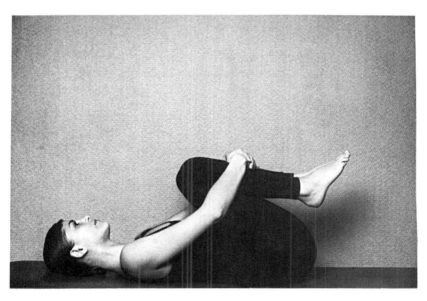

Leg Hug to Strengthen Back.

◎ Strengthen Lower Back with the Following Three Exercises:

1. Lie flat on your back with your legs extended straight in front of you. Slowly bend your knees and pull them toward your chest. Now clasp your hands on your knees and rock slowly backward and forward, hugging your knees as closely to your chest as you can. If in any position you feel tension in the part of your back where you are having difficulty, hold that position for a minute and take a deep breath and then exhale slowly while visualizing a soothing feeling penetrating the area of discomfort.

2. The Yoga cobra is often effective in relieving back pain. Lie flat on your stomach with your palms and elbows on the floor in front of you. Inhale deeply and lift your upper torso from the floor with your arms while moving your head back. As you slowly exhale, return slowly to the original position. Repeat 6 times.

3. Sit on the floor with your legs straight in front of you and your back straight. Raise your arms to shoulder height and slowly reach for your toes with your fingers. Hold for the count of three and then straighten. Repeat 6 times.

◎ Massage, Strengthen and Stretch the Upper and Middle Back with the Following Techniques:

1. Relieve upper or lower back pain by alternating ice massage with firm Circular Rhythmic Pressure. Place one or two ice cubes in a thick terry-cloth towel or wool flannel cloth or an ice bag and place directly on skin for 15 to 30 seconds. Then apply Circular Rhythmic Pressure on the area. **Caution:** Do not use ice over the kidneys or do bodywork too deeply in this area.

2. Relieve lower back pain using the Increasing Joint Motion Technique, rotating the entire leg from the hip. Do this while standing and supporting yourself against a table or the back of a chair.

3. Use the Increasing Joint Motion Technique for your shoulders. Stretch your arms out at the sides at shoulder height. Make small circles and gradually increase their size. Do 6 clockwise and 6 counterclockwise. Or: Lift your right shoulder toward your head and rotate it 6 times clockwise and 6 times counterclockwise. Now repeat with the left shoulder.

4. The trapezius muscle raises and lowers the shoulder and pulls the head backward. To release a tight trapezius, place your right hand over your right shoulder and across your back and your left hand under your left shoulder. Now try to ''hold hands.''Hold for the count of twelve. The first time you try this you may only be able to touch the tips of your index fingers. Eventually you should be able to clasp one hand in the other.

5. Relieve upper back pain using by increasing joint motion on the head and neck, shoulders and arms.

A SPECIAL NOTE ON BACK PROBLEMS

Take care of your back. Carefully reach and bend to pick up heavy objects.

Watch your posture when you are sitting, making sure that your back and spine are supported. Be aware of your posture, whether you are standing or sitting.

Use Epsom salt baths, cool to lukewarm packs, or grated fresh ginger compresses on the area of discomfort.

Rest but not excessively. This can cause atrophy of the muscles in the abdomen and lower back. Excessive rest can also lead to osteoporosis and further muscle spasms.

Use alternating hot and cold spray showers daily on areas of tension and pain.

Note: Occasionally the imbalance in the back may be so great that a back brace or orthopedic corset may be required to give adequate support to the lower thoracic and lumbar spine as well as to the abdominal muscles. This should be determined by a health professional trained in making such evaluations.

THE ABDOMEN

@ *Signs of Imbalance in the Abdomen:*

Uneven distribution of body weight when standing (greater weight on one leg or hip).

Poor posture.

Lower back pain.

Pelvis extended forward.

Digestive problems.
Flatulence and stomach cramps.
Menstrual cramps.

@ Causes of Imbalance in the Abdomen:

Tight clothes, such as girdles, tight belts, and tight jeans, tend to restrict the motion of the abdominal muscles as well as the muscles of the lower back. In addition, they affect breathing by restricting the proper action of the diaphragm. Constipation.
Tight buttocks.
Extremely tight front and back thigh muscles.
Congenital weakness.
Poor exercise habits.
Poor muscle tone in abdomen, lower back, and leg muscles.
Diseases of the abdomen, such as stomach cancer, ulcers, internal-organ (e.g., kidney, liver) malfunctions, hemorrhoids.
Gas trapped in the abdomen and rib cage.

@ Imbalances in the Digestive System

Incorrect use of back muscles, such as picking up heavy objects incorrectly.
Pregnancy.
Repressed emotions such as anger, fear, and jealousy.

@ Techniques for Relieving Abdominal Imbalances:

1. Eliminate waste and tone intestinal muscles by applying circular Pressure Point Massage to the entire abdomen in a clockwise direction, using the heel of your hand instead of your thumb. Caution: If there is acute pain, a suspected pregnancy, or any organ malfunction, do not use this technique or any other form of deep pressure.

2. Relieve gas pains and menstrual cramps by performing Muscle Rock on the abdomen.

3. Release blockages by applying light Rhythmic Pressure Point Massage on the points two inches on either side of the navel. Follow with medium Circular Pressure Point Massage on the lower back, directly behind the navel.

4. Release and soothe repressed emotions by doing relaxation and deep breathing exercises.

5. Increase bowel regularity by increasing fiber content and decreasing refined foods in your diet. Also apply gentle Vital Force Contact one inch below the navel. Apply pressure 3 times for 15 seconds each time.

6. Strengthen abdominal muscles by doing the Yoga cobra and sit ups. Lie on your back with your knees bent and your feet flat on the floor. With your hands locked at the base of your head, lift your trunk until the elbows touch your knees. Hold for the count of six. Slowly lower your back to the floor, one vertebra at a time. Repeat 6 times.

THE LEGS (HIPS, THIGHS, KNEES, AND CALVES)

◉ Signs of Imbalance in the Legs:

Tightness in front or back of thighs.
Locked knee joint.
Pain in lower back.
Very bulky, muscular thighs.
Difficulty bending knee.
Pelvic area protrudes forward.
Knock knees or bow legs.
Difficulty kneeling or sitting "Japanese style," with legs folded under the body.
Chronic pain in calf or thigh muscles.
Inability to stand for long periods of time.
Walking with a limp when there is no medical reason.
Stiffness in hip joints, particularly after sitting for a period of time.
Pain in knee. If pain is on the outside of the knee, the primary imbalance is on the inside of the thigh and shin. If the pain is on the back of the knee, the primary imbalance is probably in the calf muscles and the hamstring.

Caution: Pain under the kneecap or a knee that is unable to bend or straighten completely may be an indication of torn cartilage and may require professional attention.

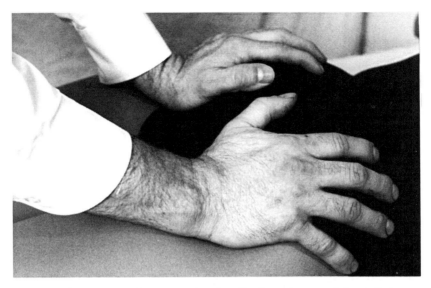

Muscle Hug on the Buttocks Can Reduce Leg and Back Pain.

@ *Causes of Imbalance in Legs:*

Congenital structural defects such as knock knees, pigeon toes, or bowed legs.

Structural imbalances such as bone spurs, calcium deposits, or excess fluid in the joints.

One leg that is shorter than the other.

Injuries to the ankle, the most common being a sprain.

Overweight.

Pregnancy.

@ *Specific Leg and Knee Injuries*

Shin splints. These can result from either the tearing of a membrane between the two shin bones or the tearing of a muscle in the shins.

Arthritic conditions of the knees and legs.

"Housewife's knee" results from a constant bruising from kneeling over a long period of time that irritates the bursas under the knee. This can be prevented by wearing knee pads.

"Football Knee." These are meniscus injuries involving trauma to the crescent-shaped cartilage found in the knee joint. This type of injury is most commonly found in football players, which is the source of its name. Other causes are a blow to the outside of the knee or a forced sideways bending of the knee joint (which the knee is not designed for) caused by stepping in a hole or any motion that turns the ankle.

Caution: All meniscus injuries should receive professional attention; however, the techniques in this section for healing knee imbalances can be very helpful.

@ *Techniques for Relieving Leg Imbalances:*

1. Preventing shin splints. Apply deep Circular and General Pressure Point Massage on the soft tissue that lies between the two lower leg bones. Increasing Joint Motion Technique on ankle, moving the foot up and down 36 times.

2. Correcting shin splints:

Sit with the painful leg elevated as much as possible.

Apply Circular Pressure Massage on the shin.

Rub an ice bag up and down shins. Do this for 5 minutes on and 5 minutes off. Do 6 alternating cycles of ice massage (30 minutes).

3. Relax tight muscles, relieve congested muscles, and increase circulation for the entire leg.

By using the palm to apply deep Pressure Point Massage. Do this by working the palm of the hand down the entire leg, working on the front, back and side of the thigh and the back and side of the calf.

Follow with Muscle Kneading on the entire leg, working on the front, back, and side of the thigh and the back and side of the calf. **Note:** It is important that you do not put pressure on the shin bone or the knee.

4. Release restricted Chi in the lower leg by applying the Polarity Similars Technique.

First place your index finger on the shoulder and the middle finger of your other hand on the hip.

Place your index finger on the elbow and the middle finger of your other hand on the knee.

5. Release restricted Chi in the thigh by using the Gravity Rock Technique. Place one hand on any tender point about one half to one inch on the inside of the pelvic bone. With the other hand, grasp the thigh firmly, without squeezing too hard, and begin to rock thigh muscles from side to side while pressing firmly but not too deeply on pelvic point.

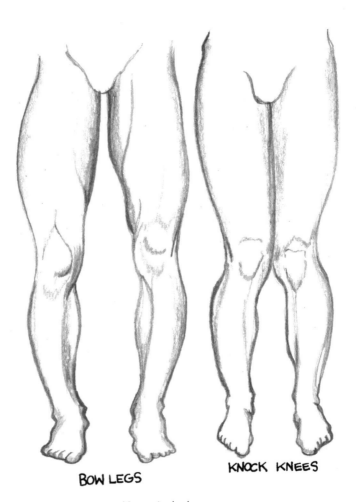

BOW LEGS   KNOCK KNEES

Knee Imbalances.

◉ *After an Injury, Use the Following Methods to Strengthen the Knee:*

For the first twenty-four hours, use an elastic brace on the knee whenever leg is in use. However, try to stay off the leg as much as possible.

For most minor injuries to the knee, apply cold water or ice packs for twenty-four hours, stay off the leg, and elevate the knee. When using ice or cold water packs, apply for twenty minutes and then remove for fifteen, After ice packs have been used for twenty-four hours, apply warm castor-oil packs.*

Strengthen the quadriceps muscles by flexing or contracting the thigh muscle against the resistance of the hand. This quadriceps is the muscle which stabilize the knees.

Apply arnica lotion right after the strain or injury takes place. This herbal lotion is available in health food stores.

Many knee injuries incurred today are the result of poor running and jogging habits, the worst of which is wearing poorly designed and poorly fitted shoes. To prevent knee injuries, if you run or jog, even occasionally, you should invest in a good pair of runner's shoes. Runners with knee problems should not exert any pressure on the knee or do exercises that cause you to bend your leg.

◉ *Strengthen the Calf Muscles and the Achilles Tendon:*

Lying on your back, increasing Joint Range of Motion with your foot. Lift the foot 5 to 10 inches off the floor and rotate it 6 times clockwise and 6 times counterclockwise.

Stand approximately 3 feet from a wall, facing it, and rest your hands on the wall. Make certain that your body is on an angle. Now slowly raise your heels until you are standing on your toes. Hold this position for a count of twenty and then slowly lower your heels to the ground. Repeat 3 times.

Do the Gravity Rock, followed by Circular Pressure Point Massage on your calf.

◉ *Flower Remedies*

When the legs are weak and out of balance, it may indicate that a person may have reached the limits of their endurance. For

---

*Some people have reported positive results from DMSO, a waste product of the wood pulp industry. There have been claims of therapeutic benefit from its use, particularly in cases where surgery seemed to be the only course of action.

those moments of deep despair, when the anguish seems to be unbearable, Sweet Chestnut is the flower remedy of choice.

THE ANKLES AND FEET

@ *Healing of Imbalances of the Feet Has Four Primary Goals:*

1. To improve circulation around the feet.
2. To stabilize the position of the feet in relation to the legs so that the body is correctly balanced.
3. To create a full range of motion for all joints of the foot.
4. To strengthen the supporting muscles in the foot.

FEET

Most imbalances in the feet result from the burden of body weight. Improper posture and ill-fitting shoes also cause problems. For proper posture, body weight is spread equally between both feet. The most weight is borne by the heel bone (calcaneus). The remainder rests on the outer arch of the foot and metatarsal bones.

@ *Signs of Imbalance in the Ankles and Feet:*

High instep (high arch).

Flat feet (fallen arches). People with this imbalance usually wear out the inner edges of the soles of their shoes.

Feet turned extremely in or out, "pigeon toed" or "slew-footed." (Slew-footedness, excessive turnout of the foot and ankle, and the resultant tension in the foot, ankle, and knee, is commonly experienced by ballet dancers who have been improperly trained.)

Hip problems.

Hammer toe, a condition in which the first bone of the toe points upward while the second and third bones point downward.

Toe joints that are constantly flexed, usually due to tension and contracted hamstrings.

Extreme sensitivity to touch. This may be experienced as ticklish-ness, pain, or a general dislike of having the feet touched.

◉ *Causes of Imbalance in the Ankles and Feet:*

A rotated pelvis. This may result in fallen arches.

Poorly fitted or pointed shoes. These may cause the ligaments to shorten, the joint capsules to contract, adhesions to form where they should not be, and an increasingly rigid longitudinal arch that can affect the structural balance of the entire body. More often than not, misshaped toes are due to poor shoe choice over the years.

Standing on your feet for extended periods of time.

Tightness of inner-thigh and lower-back muscles may result in fallen arches, although in many cases, fallen arches are congenital.

High insteps. This places the body's center of gravity in the wrong place, and can cause extensive postural problems.

Compression of the nerve against the thighbone, crossing the legs, and wearing high heels can contribute to a condition known as "dropped foot." This is an abnormal extension, or movement of the top of the foot away from the shinbone. When a person is wearing high heels, the foot is in a state of abnormal extension (or plantar flexion).

Poor posture when walking.

◉ *Techniques for Relieving Ankle and Foot Imbalances:*

◉ *To Heal Injured Feet*

1. Tap the bottom of the feet with fingertips in a very rapid motion. This has a tonifying effect.

2. Use the Increasing Joint Motion Technique on feet. Rotate each foot 12 times clockwise and counterclockwise.

3. Muscle Hug the feet and the calves.

4. Use light Pressure Point Massage along the outsides of the feet.

5. Flex the foot 3 times toward the shinbone and 3 times downward (away from shinbone).

6. Soak the ankles and feet in warm water with Epsom salts or sea salt.

7. Apply Polarity Similars Contacts on ankles and wrists; toes and fingers.

8. The Increasing Joint Motion Technique on toes. Grasp the tip of each toe and rotate clockwise 3 times and counterclockwise 3 times.

9. Twice a day, elevate the feet for 5 to 10 minutes.

@ To Help Correct a Sprained Ankle, after First Aid Has Been Applied

1. After the sprain, apply an ice bag or a cold-water compress. Apply ice for 15 minutes of every hour. Resting the area in between these periods. Continue for 24 hours.

2. After 24 hours, while in a sitting position move the joint through its normal range of motion. Use only up-and-down movements in the beginning. Lift your sprained ankle from the floor about twelve inches and then slowly point your toe down and then up. Proceed through this movement 6 times. Repeat several times a day. After this, you can begin to do a circular range of motion.

3. Whenever possible revitalize the area by elevating the foot.

4. Twenty-four hours after the sprain, soak your foot in a warm solution of Epsom salts.

5. When the pain and swelling begin to subside, apply Circular Pressure Point Massage to the entire area around the ankle.

6. After two or three days, while standing, lift the right heel slowly and shift the weight to the left foot. Then slowly lift your right heel and shift your weight to the right foot while lowering it to the floor. Keep your toes on the floor at all times. Repeat 6 times for each foot.

HYPERTENSION, IMPOTENCE, EMOTIONAL TRAUMA

In addition to relieving the musculoskeletal imbalances, Shaman Massage and healing techniques have proved to be beneficial in other common types of imbalances, three of which are hypertension (high blood pressure), impotence and general tension.

HYPERTENSION

Hypertension is often related to poor nutritional patterns, emotional stress, spiritual pain, or lack of exercise. Overeating, too much refined sugar, too much salt in the diet, excessive smoking, excessive alcohol consumption, poor emotional disposition, and kidney dysfunction can all contribute to hypertension. In addition to changing your eating patterns and developing a consistent exercise and movement program, visualization techniques can help balance your Chi with a resulting reduction in blood pressure. I use a gentle Gravity Rock on the stomach area to balance the kidneys, These will help soothe and relax the nervous system and revitalize the vital organs.

IMPOTENCE

Most men experience impotence at some time in their lives. It can result from physical and emotional imbalances or a combination of both. Recent research indicates that in as much as fifty percent of all cases, impotence is caused by emotional factors. When the causes are physical, it is often the use of medication, including those that are often prescribed for hypertension, that are the source of the problem. Whether the problem is physical or psychological, Shamanic breathing and deep visualization can free the energy pathways of the effects of fear, worry, hate, and jealousy. Use movement techniques that help to energize and revitalize the system, such as head stands, shoulder stands, or the use of a slant board for at least five minutes a day.

General imbalances in Chi can manifest in the body as premature ejaculation, loss of erection, frigidity, and diminished sexual drive. These may be corrected through herbal healing. Palmetto berries, damiana, pumpkin seeds, and foods high in zinc and vitamin E may all help. Exercises designed to strengthen the lower back and abdominal muscles can also be helpful. To stimulate the sexual organs, directly apply The Chi Balancing Technique to the point about one inch below the navel several times a day.
Note: These recommendations will not increase sexual potency in individuals who already are functioning at their optimal level.

BODYWORKS*

	A	B	C	D
Allergies	6, 7, 8, 36			
Ankle pain	10, 11, 12			
Arm pain	14	33		88, 89, 90
Arthritis	2, 4, 5	13, 26, 16		89, 90
Asthma	17, 19, 18, 20			91
Bronchitis	14, 6, 18		21	92, 74
Bursitis	21, 14		39, 23	88
Calf pain	4, 24			
Cold	7, 25, 8, 17, 18	26	73, 27, 28	
Colitis	3, 31	40	29, 27, 30	
Constipation	32, 3, 31, 11, 9	26, 33, 93		92
Cough	34, 75, 36, 17, 11		57, 27	94
Cystitis	15, 31		29, 37, 70	
Dental pain			38, 39	
Diarrhea	3, 2, 31	26, 40	27, 54	68
Dizziness			58, 42	
Elbow pain	14	26, 43	23	62
Fatigue	14		45, 23, 41	
Sore eyes	48	26	54	73
Facial pain		26, 78	50, 51	
Foot pain	12, 36, 11	87, 80, 52, 16	51	76
Foot pain	11	52	51	
Gallbladder		52	30, 29	
Gastritis	3, 17, 2, 53		44	
Gingivitis		26	50, 35	
Gout			54, 55	
Hand pain			23, 44	
Hayfever		26	57, 28	56
Headache	8		27, 21, 58, 59, 57, 26	
Hiccups	2, 5, 21		29	
High blood pressure	2		60	61
Indigestion	12, 9, 3		30	62
Influenza	11, 6		57	63

*See Charts A, B, C, and D (pp. 252-255).

BODYWORKS

	A	B	C	D
Insomnia	11	64, 65		61
Knee pain	15, 5			
Leg pain	4, 32, 5, 15	53, 40, 65		
Low blood pressure		66	28	
Lower back pain	24	16	51	67
Menstrual irregularity	11		37	68, 70
Menstrual pain		66	70	21, 71
Stress (mental)	20		42, 28, 21, 57	
Migraine headache		26, 72, 64	37, 21, 38, 28, 3	73
Motion sick-ness	2, 21	75	42	74
Nasal conges-tion	17, 8, 7, 12		42	
Nausea	2, 5, 11, 72, 9		29, 27	68
Neck pain	17, 12	64, 72	44	73
Sciatica	32, 4	16	74, 51	75, 76
Shoulder pain		43	23, 44, 45	
Sinus prob-lems	77, 7	26, 78	42	56
Sore throat		26	35	
Stiff neck		78, 79, 80	28, 23	73
Stomach pain	75	40	30, 29, 37	81, 72
Tennis elbow		26, 43	44	82
Tinnitus	8	83, 85, 26		61
Tonsillitis	5	26, 87, 78		86
Toothache	77	16, 33, 64, 83		
Whiplash	19, 8	26	44, 57	
Earache		26		
Fainting			38	71
Hemorrhage	14, 36			63
Testicle pain				68
Wound pain		87	23, 69	
Reducing hunger		83		

EMOTIONAL TRAUMA

◉ Indicators of Emotional Trauma:

Backaches.
Tight shoulders.
Headache.
Insomnia.
Grinding of teeth (bruxism).
Furrowed eyebrows and/or lines on forehead.
Squinting eyes.

◉ Causes of Tension:

Poor posture. Incorrect body alignment places undue stress on all parts of the body.

Stressful occupation. Tension at the work place can accumulate and lead to physical illness.

Nutritional deficiencies. Diet deficient in essential vitamins and minerals.

No outlet for emotional expression. All work and no play does more than make Jack or Jane dull.

Poor movement and exercise patterns.

Poor sleeping habits. The cause can be too many pillows, an improper mattress, street noises, ingestion of a heavy meal or snacks at bedtime, and not enough fresh air. Lack of certain vitamins, especially B6, may prevent the achievement of certain brain rhythms so that the deep sleep period is not entered.

◉ Techniques to Relieve Emotional Trauma:

1. Apply Pressure Point Massage to the back of the head using the flat area of the thumbs. Begin at the back of the head where it meets the neck (occiput area). Gently press this area from left to right, then from right to left. Apply pressure to the entire surface at least 3 times before moving to the next area.

2. Knead the ears. Place the earlobe between the thumb and the index finger and with a rubbing motion, softly squeeze. Repeat several times on each ear.

3. Gravity Rock the stomach. Your partner should lie flat on his back. Place your right hand on the lower abdomen and your left

hand gently on the abdomen. Rock the stomach with a gentle back and forth motion.

    4. Apply Pressure Point Massage to the feet.

    5. Gravity Rock the back.

    6. Complete the energy release by using visualization techniques. Ask your partner to lie flat on his back. Have him close his eyes. Slowly, take a deep, slow breath. Inhale, hold it, and release. Repeat this 3 times.

◉ Energy Balancing Visualization

Step 1
Visualize a soft blue sky with white fluffy clouds gently passing overhead.

Step 2
Let your entire body go limp. Take the tension first from your feet by contracting the muscles. Now totally release and relax. Repeat this process.

Step 3
Focus on tensing and releasing the front and back leg muscles. Repeat this 3 times, tensing then releasing.

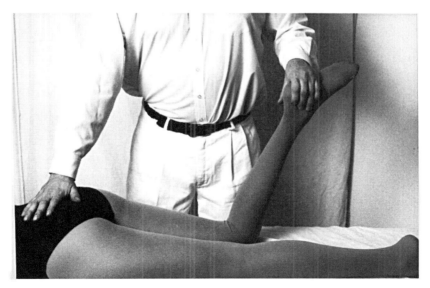

Polarity Similars: Sacrum to Heel for Emotional Trauma.

Step 4
Shrug your shoulders, then make a fist, and then release and relax both.

Step 5
Finally tense the face, pucker the lips, tightly close the eyes, and then release, relax and release. Now take another deep breath and exhale, allowing your body to completely relax.

HANDS-ON HEALING AND SHAMAN MASSAGE TECHNIQUE

@ *Skin Rolling*

This is a powerful technique for freeing up emotional trauma. Among Mongolian Shamans it is a common belief that muscles "remember" early fears, traumas and painful experiences. The traumas, and the muscular tensions they create, remain intimately linked until they are released from the body through careful, skilled manipulation. It is thought by many teachers that each type of fear is stored in a different part of the body. For example, fear of loss would be stored in the lower back; of being overburdened would be stored in the upper back and shoulders; worries and expectations in the scalp; thoughts of inadequacy in the thighs. Rolling each area, opens the way for positive emotions and feelings of love.

It is essential, in practicing effective Shaman massage, that trapped Chi be released from the points at which the tendons attach them to the bone. When this is done the body will operate more freely, with the muscles and bones working in alignment rather than against each other. This is commonly called breaking through the body armor. Among the benefits to be achieved by using skin rolling in combination with Circular Pressure Point Massage are:

- a shift in body structure
- reduction of old stress patterns
- creation of new postural patterns postures

Step 1
Take the skin and and place it between your thumb and your index and middle finger.

Step 2
Lift it gently and begin to roll it in long, vertical strokes.

Note: This technique will be easy in some areas of your body but in other areas the skin will not release from the underlying tissue. As you continue to practice this technique, the skin will release. In time this technique will open certain doors for emotional expression and free up the emotional memory. The physical benefits of skin rolling include increased circulation, greater elasticity to the skin, and a more youthful appearance.

⊚ *Flower Remedy*

Skin rolling is especially valuable for those who, for no apparent reason, have resigned themselves to their circumstances. Having become indifferent, little effort is made to improve things or find joy. The flower remedy, Wild Rose, has an expansive effect on the emotions which is well suited for those who respond to skin rolling.

HEALING HANDS TECHNIQUES

⊚ *Connective Tissue De-armoring*

This technique is a combination of Skin Rolling and Deep Pressure Point Massage using oils and sliding the finger pressure sideways (tranverse) across the muscle fibers. It is a very effective tool to reduce body armoring and free up emotional energy stored in muscle and connective tissue.

Remember:
1. The massage should be given transverely.
2. This will free the ligament to move in its normal way over bone.
3. This may help to smooth off a rough, scarred tendon surface.
4. The thicker and stronger the tissue to be worked on, the more tranverse finger pressure is required.

The goal in all transverse movement is to reduce the formation of adhering scar tissue fibers.

The only limiting factors are the size of the area to be worked and the elasticity of the underlying skin. When deep transverse movement is required, the most effective approach is a sliding

Pressure Point Massage in a straight transverse movement, as opposed to Circular Pressure Point Massage or a stationary deep pressure.

◉ To Apply the Connective Tissue De-armoring Technique

1. Find correct spot.
2. Apply contact properly.
3. In lesions, always work in a transverse motion.
4. The movement must be deep.
5. Client must be in a comfortable and suitable position.
6. Muscle must be relaxed while technique is applied.

After the session, contract (as much as possible) the joint and muscle area that has been worked on. This contraction should be done in a non-weight-bearing position.

The more recent the injury, the more important it is that you do not put too much strain on the area. Exercises against resistance are to be avoided till healing takes place.

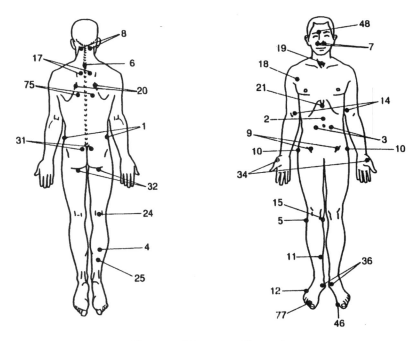

Shaman Massage Chart A.

When correcting a lesion, it is not the deep contact which is of greatest importance but the intensity of the transverse motion which will have the greatest effect.

Note: Pain of injury should not be confused with pain from the session. Often, if a session involves great discomfort and deep pressure, the area worked on will become very tender. This tenderness may remain even days after the completion of the session. It is important to be able to determine the difference between the pain of the session and the pain from the injury being treated. To do so is a basic process. Simply stretch passively the treated area and contract the area against light resistance. If there is no pain in movement under this test, then treatment is completed.

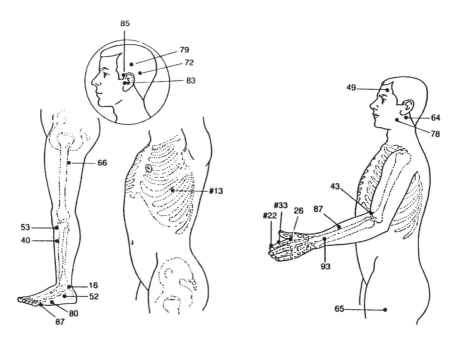

Shaman Massage Chart B.

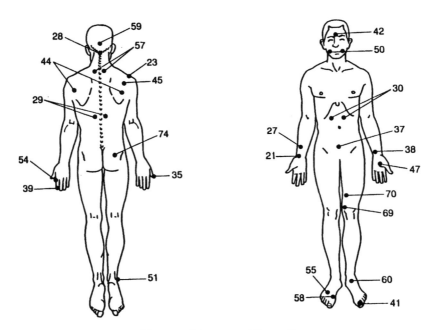

Shaman Massage Chart C.

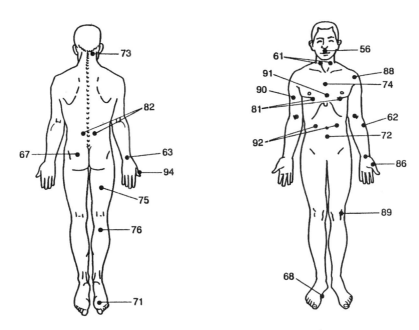

Shaman Massage Chart D.

CHAPTER 11

@

HEALING THROUGH MOVEMENT

Hands-On Healing and Shaman Massage are forms of passive exercise. Active exercise adds an entirely new component to this work. Freedom of movement is one of the keys to physical and emotional health. For creating and maintaining emotional health, movement can be a source for unlimited creativity. It is a natural response to music and is a key means for expression. Physiologically, movement acts as a pumping mechanism for the body, initiating the exchange of essential fluids at all levels of the organism.

When we are babies, our bodies are soft and pliable. Body unity is already there. It isn't something you have to develop, create, or form. The various systems of the body are not distinct other than in how we view them. Fascia, muscles, bones and nerves are all intricately connected.

We respond to stimuli with a large range of physical motions as we bounce back quickly from physical and emotional stress. As we leave childhood, our physical movements are defined more and more by societal pressures, organization, and "accepted" images that are imposed on us through television and other media images. These factors limit the development of our full physical, emotional and spiritual potential and help establish rigid patterns of thought, action and feeling.

Two key factors in the development of our body structures are our need to have approval of our appearance and our need to feel safe. In our desire to avoid physical and emotional pain, we use posture and movement styles that may create approval from others, but may also create structural problems.

In a complex and somewhat surreal series of events, we find ourselves acting in ways that we expect others to approve of. Others see these actions and respond to them. We then respond to their response to our actions and so on and so forth. After a while we are so detached from our true nature that we lose touch with our feelings and any sense of self-knowledge. This detachment from self causes physical rigidity, fear, confusion and various structural and muscular problems. In order to shift the way we act, it is essential that we make a distinction between our physical body and the "social body" that influences us. Once we make this distinction, we change our self-image and the motivations tied to it. The more conscious we are of our actions, the greater our potential for freeing ourselves from habitual patterns of thought and action. This freedom enables us to expand our emotional and physical capabilities. Movement is a valuable medium in which to create this shift and is an important key to the nervous system and to all our actions, thoughts, and feelings. The role of the myofascial system in the freedom or limitation of movement is an interesting one.

When the embryo is still in the womb, individual muscle fibers form in a matrix of fascia. This appears as a single fascial sheath. As time passes, and you change spiritually, emotionally and physically, the fascia changes as well. If you were to break your arm, for example, the fascia around the healed bone would become thick, tough and stringy. This "lesion" or "knot" can be felt when you massage and poke around the area. Lesions of this type will limit the normal range of motion in neighboring muscles by shortening the fascial planes and creating adhesions between fascia, muscles and bones. This can be the foundation for physical and emotional dis-ease by limiting body movement and the flow of essential fluids through the flesh. Even weight lifting and strength building, if not accompanied by stretching and proper postural training, will contribute to these problems. In extreme physical and emotional blocks, the fascial covering of one muscle group may become enmeshed with the fascia of another group, resulting in restricted movement through the area and limited emotional expression and self-awareness. Many people live with various medical problems that are asymptomatic or are never properly diagnosed but which cause energetic and structural blockages in the system. For example, there have been people who suffered with undiagnosed polio. This deeply affected the fascia and the associated psoas muscles by limiting movement and balance in the pelvis and legs. Yet no one would ever know the source of the problem. Any trauma to the system, whether physical or emotional, can cause structural shifts by influencing the fascial plane.

@ Posture

The way you walk, stand, and sit serves as a mirror of what is happening to your body and can also be a source for energy imbalances. Remember that what happens to one area of your body influences other areas in ways that might not be obvious at first. Posture is actually the physical manifestation of your emotions, muscles, ligaments, tendons, bones, circulation, and flexibility combined. When you become conscious of posture you begin to see that if your sacrum bones shift in one direction, the cranial bones will respond. When your ankles become weak in a particular way, the hips and jaw bone will respond. Standing and walking with the weight improperly balanced can contribute to lower back pain. Rounded shoulders can cause problems in the thighs, legs, and feet. When you are posturally integrated, you look better and feel better.

Upright posture demands specific strength and balance between your major antigravity muscles—the erector spinae (these run along your spine), quadriceps (your upper thigh muscles) and gastrocnemius (your calf muscles).

Your posture is also an accurate mirror of stress. When improper use of the body is undertaken before there is psychological, vibrational (balancing in the Chakras) and physiological readiness to respond to a stressful activity, the body will assume faulty patterns.

Breath and visualization exercises can balance out energetic distortions, while movement reeducation and structurally based exercises are designed to affect the muscles and joints and heal injuries. It is in this way that the healing power is manifested through movement.

By using one's body with maximum efficiency, fatigue, pain and strain can be avoided, tasks made easier and safer, and better results achieved. As mentioned before, improving the posture, adopting sensible lifting positions, and exercising or massaging stiff muscles and joints all can be very effective for eliminating the stresses and strains put upon the spine.

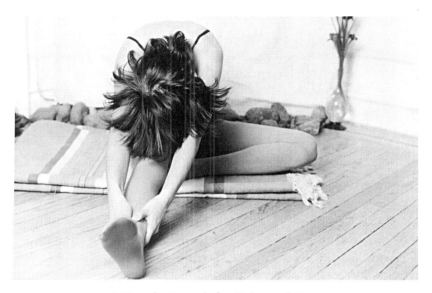

A Simple Stretch for Balanced Posture.

@ *Healing Movement Is More Than Exercise*

When people think of exercise they often refer to building muscles or increasing muscle tone. Though we generally think about the outer muscles of the body, it is important to keep in mind that there are muscles throughout the body that cannot be strengthened or stretched simply by performing typical exercise.

Structured body movement has been recognized for centuries as essential for good physical and spiritual well-being. Throughout time, cultures as diverse as those of the Greeks, Romans, Egyptians, Indians, and Chinese have used techniques designed to enhance not just physical but moral and emotional development. Effective movement usually involves self-propelled movement or resistance by the muscles to a fixed point (as in isometrics). In the process of massage there is no self-propelled movement. All movement is carried out by the therapist without resistance or assistance of the patient.

Energy-based bodywork bridges exercise and massage as the individual becomes more involved in his own healing through guided movements that are integrated into the bodywork session. In the end the goal remains the same: to balance the vibrational and energy centers, increase circulation, joint range of movement and create a greater sense of wholeness and well-being. Massage, energy healing, guided movement and exercise go hand in hand. Though healing touch can relieve tension and pain, guided movement combined with effective breathing can do the same.

Part of the amazing balance between touch and movement is that healing touch can even relieve the soreness and tightness that can result from exercise, just as proper movement enhances the effect of massage by improving muscle tone, circulation, and posture. Even the best massages, given frequently and consistently, cannot substitute for proper movement, integrated breathing and the healing touch.

Exercise and movement reeducation are not luxuries when it comes to being healthy. You require exercise in order to function at your best. Most people assume that exercise involves stretching, aerobics and strength building. In healing touch and Shaman massage, exercise and movement are as much part of the movement of consciousness as it is movement of the body.

@ Are You Exercise-Deficient? Use the Following Checklist:

- suffer frequent headaches
- sleep poorly, have difficulty going to sleep, or wake up tired
- back pains
- overweight
- difficulty remembering important things
- underweight
- tire easily
- irritable outbursts
- depressed and moody
- low interest in sex
- body full of tension, aches, and pains that don't seem to have any physical basis
- shallow and drained complexion

If you have five of the above twelve symptoms, it is important that you integrate greater amounts of healing movement in your daily life-style.

@ *Healing Through Movement*

An effective program of movement for increasing your healing powers should be enjoyable, fun and empowering. This approach integrates a combination of visualization, stretching, toning, bending, and aerobics. These will increase strength, expand flexibility in the joints, increase circulation, strengthen the heart, center and focus the mind, bring a glow to the complexion, improve posture, and promote an emotional flow by freeing up body armoring in the connective tissue.

The commitment to this program requires about 30 minutes in the morning (time focused on physical movement), and 10 minutes before bed: this time is focused on quiet contemplation. It is more effective to practice intense physical movement and exercise in the morning; in the evening, it may be overstimulating to the system.

The combination of the morning and evening sections of the program will coordinate body and mind and produce greater feelings of peace, harmony, grace, and poise.

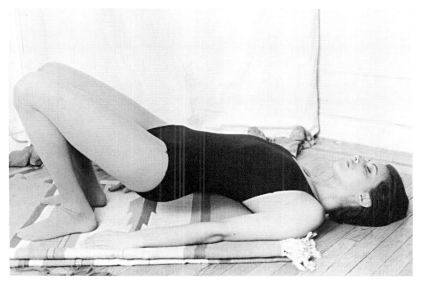

Pelvic Lift for Concentrating Chi.

◉ *Here Are Some Basic Guidelines for Concentrating Your Chi and Freeing Shamanic Energy Centers:*

1. As you put together your movement and exercise program, develop a consistent pattern of dance and movement. Dedicate a specific time and place daily.

2. Exercise in a well-ventilated room, preferably one where there is fresh air circulating.

3. Keep your foods simple. Fruits, vegetables, broth, etc. To avoid digestive problems do not eat a heavy meal for an hour before or after doing the movements.

4. Wear loose-fitting, natural-fiber clothing.

5. If you are going to sweat heavily, wear the type of material that allows sweat to evaporate. This is especially important for women, in order to reduce yeast and other types of vaginal infections.

6. If your movements are to be done on a floor, use a mat or a folded blanket.

7. Be gentle with yourself. Do not force your body into uncomfortable positions.

8. Enter each movement gradually and slowly, never bending suddenly or bouncing into a pose or position. Bouncing or quick movements do not stretch out a muscle, they strain it. Strong sustained pull or pressure has a stretching effect.

9. When each movement is completed, breathe fully and allow your body to relax for a few moments.

10. While performing the movements, focus your breathing and mind on specific tensions and blocks and visualize them leaving your body through exhalation.

11. As you gain mastery, gradually increase the difficulty, range of motion, number of repetitions, and fluidity of the exercises and integrate them with self-massage, breathing, music and prayer.

The movements presented here are designed to increase range of motion and tone, improve circulation; increase or release blocked up energy and create a balance for the entire myofascial system.

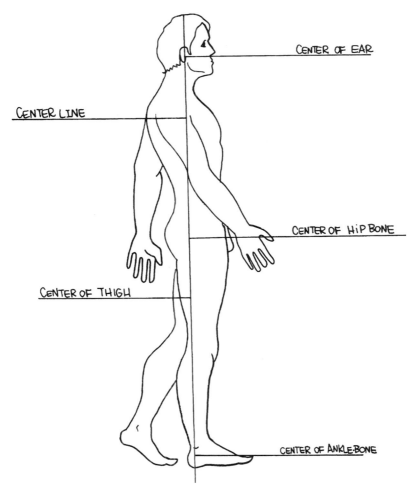

CENTER OF EAR

CENTER LINE

CENTER OF HIP BONE

CENTER OF THIGH

CENTER OF ANKLE-BONE

Perfect Posture.

THE SHAMAN'S DAILY MOVEMENT PROGRAM

@ *Body Shake*

The body shake is a basic preparatory movement that is done prior to the rest of the movement program. It is stimulating for the circulation and can bring an energized sense to the entire body. It is a wonderful movement for combatting depression by ridding the body of tension and negative emotions.

@ *How to Begin the Body Shake*

Standing tall and starting with your feet, shake each part of your body. The sequence goes in the following order:

Shake your feet, your ankles, the legs, the hips, and the waist, followed by the shoulders, arms and hands, neck, and head.

@ *Body Stretch*

The purpose of this movement is to strengthen the Achilles tendon, heart, hamstrings, and the shoulders. It is also a valuable tool for reducing insomnia.

Step 1
Stand tall and raise your arms above your head.

Step 2
Stretch your arms and fingers as if you were reaching for the stars and clawing the air.

Step 3
As you reach, inhale deeply through your nose while rising onto your toes. Now exhale slowly.

Step 4
Gradually return to your starting position, with your arms hanging loosely at your sides.

Step 5
Repeat Steps 1 through 4 at least 3 times.

After you have mastered this exercise, increase the difficulty by doing it with your eyes closed.

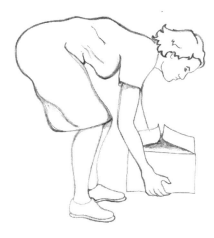

Lifting Incorrectly.

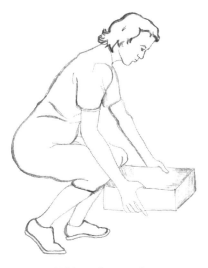

Lifting Correctly.

◉ *Body Bend*

The body bend is useful for strengthening the lower back and abdominal muscles.

Step 1
Standing tall, loosely bend from the waist, slowly dropping your head and arms.

Step 2
Take a long slow breath through your mouth. This will have the effect of automatically lifting your torso.

Step 3
Exhale slowly. This will automatically lower your torso and bring your fingers closer to your toes.

Step 4
Inhale and exhale 3 times.

Caution: If you feel pain behind your knees, bend over only as far as is comfortable or stop the exercise altogether.

Now exhale, and as you do so draw your legs even closer to your chest. Inhale and exhale 3 times. Slowly straighten your legs and lower them to the floor.

@ *Leg Lift*

The leg lift is valuable in strengthening the lower back and abdominal muscles and for stretching the thigh muscles.

Step 1
Lie flat on your back.

Step 2
Lift your legs off the floor about three feet.

Step 3
Inhale deeply as you are raising your legs. Hold them in this position as long as you can while holding your breath.

Step 4
Exhale slowly while slowly lowering your legs. Perform this movement 3 times. After you have mastered this exercise, increase the difficulty by not lifting your legs as high. This will create more tension in your abdominal and back muscles.

@ *Feet Over Head*

This movement tonifies the entire system and releases blocked Chi in the legs, hips, and lower back muscles.

As the involved muscles begin to stretch and strengthen, you will be able to put your feet farther and farther back.

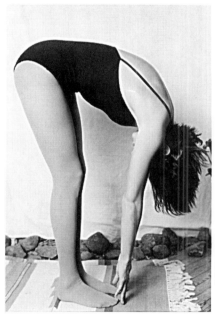

Body Bend.

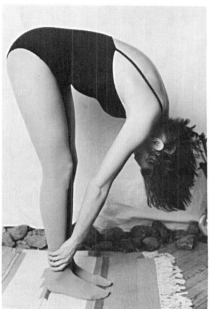

Body Bend.

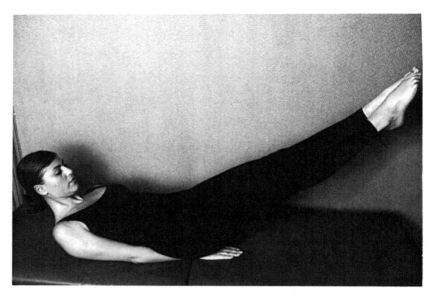

Leg Extension to Strengthen Back.

Step 1
Lie flat on your back and take three long deep breaths.

Step 2
Lift your legs off the floor, and try to touch your feet to the floor behind your head.

Step 3
If you can't go all the way back, just take your legs as far as you can without forcing them.

Step 4
Hold for the count of ten and then bring them back down.

@ *Cobra*

This movement stimulates blood flow, tonifies the internal organs, and strengthens the buttocks and chest muscles.

Step 1
As you lie on your stomach bend your elbows and place your hands at the sides of your chest.

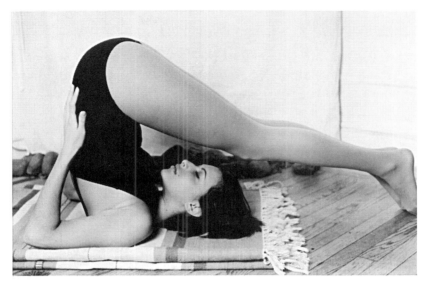

Feet Over Head.

Step 2

Raise your chest and feet at the same time. Repeat 3 times.

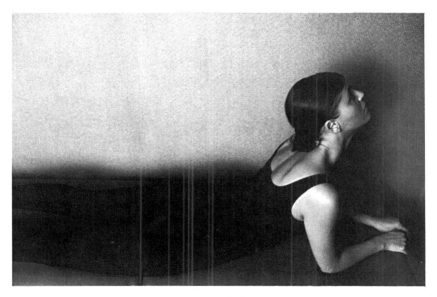

Yoga Cobra.

@ *Indian Style Posture (The Folding Lotus))*

This classic posture, thousands of years old and used by Shamans, healers and yogis, will aid digestion and balance Chi in the liver, colon, and heart.

Step 1
Sit on the floor with your back straight.

Step 2
Cross your legs at the ankles and try to place knees flat on the floor. Don't be discouraged if you can't lay them flat at once. With daily practice you will soon be able to.

Step 3
Now cross your arms and place your hands on the opposite knees.

Step 4
While in this position, slowly bend from the waist and lower your head as close to the floor as you can. Hold for the count of five.

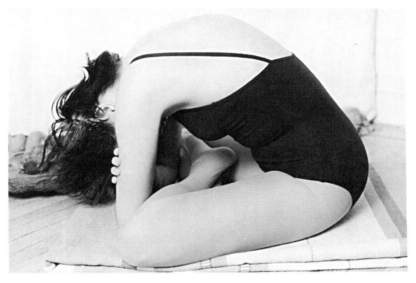

Indian Style Sit.

@ Seiza (Traditional Japanese Sitting Posture)

This classic seiza posture will balance Chi in the abdominal and pelvic area. It is used in some Tantric traditions to improve sexual functioning.

Step 1
Kneel on the floor with your legs tucked under you.

Step 2
Try to sit on the floor between your heels.

Step 3
Slowly lean back, first resting your hands, then your wrists, then your elbows, then your shoulders on the floor, and ending with your arms straight at your sides. Stop at whatever point you begin to feel discomfort and hold for the count of ten.

Step 4
Slowly return to the starting position.

@ Riding the Horse

This movement strengthens shins, thighs, and abdomen.

Step 1
Stand tall, feet together.

Step 2
Now move your right foot to the right about 2 feet.

Step 3
Point your toes outward at about a 45-degree angle.

Step 4
Holding your back very straight, bend your knees as deep as you can. Hold for the count of five.

@ Pulling The Bow

This movement will strengthen fingers, arms, shoulders, upper back, and neck.

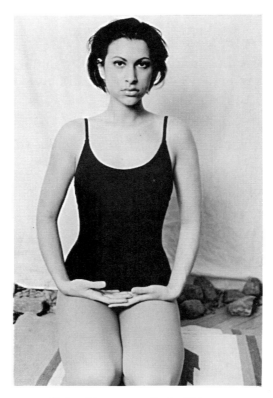

Seiza (Japanese Style Sit).

Step 1
Get into the Riding a Horse position.

Step 2
Raise your arms slowly above your knees.

Step 3
Now, as if to pull a bow, extend your right arm across your body, with your right fingers open and spread, and your left hand in a fist.

Step 4
With your left hand stable on the bow, slowly pull your right hand back as if pulling the string, clenching your fist as you go.

Step 5
As you pull your right arm back behind your right shoulder, turn your head to the right, ending with your right arm stretched behind you.

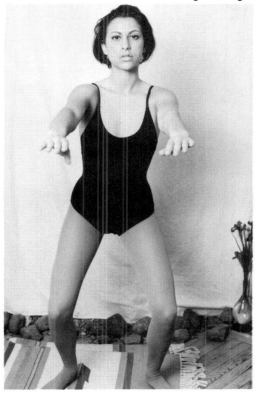

Riding the Horse.

Step 6
Slowly lower your arms. Then raise them again and do the exercise in the opposite direction.

@ Foot Rotation

The movement strengthens the toe, foot, and ankle muscles.

Step 1
Standing tall, lift one foot about twelve inches from the floor.

Step 2
Flex the foot up and down, 6 times in each direction.

Step 3
Rotate the foot, 12 times clockwise and 12 times counterclockwise.

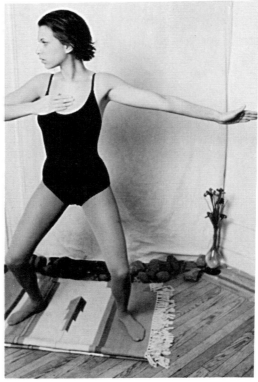

Pulling the Bow.

Step 4
Repeat for the other foot.

@ Aerobics

Aerobics stimulates circulation and energizes the total system.

1. Now stretch whatever part of your body feels stiff and knotty. Be creative.

2. Run in place to a count of 200, gradually increasing to 500;
   or
   walk fast (race walk) for 30 minutes, 3 times per week;
   or
   dance vigorously for at least 5 minutes to your favorite up-tempo record, being as creative as you can, engaging your whole body, and constantly moving.

◎ Gravity Reversal

The shoulder stand is a powerful movement to clear the mind, stimulate internal organs, and purify the blood. In Yoga it is considered balancing for the thyroid, digestion, nervousness, sinuses, sexual strength, hair, and eyesight.

Do a shoulder stand for 5 minutes. Gravity reversal techniques help to stretch the spine and increase blood flow to the head and upper extremities. The result of this is reduced stress and a greater sense of health and well-being.

◎ Bringing It All Together

This meditation will induce a feeling of peace, harmony, and tranquility.

Now you can begin your day with the feeling that you are able to do whatever it is that needs to be done.

Step 1
Lie flat on your back with your eyes closed.

Step 2
Visualize a snow-covered mountain, the ocean, or any natural sea or a landscape that makes you feel very good.

Step 3
Inhale, long and slow, and experience the energy flowing through your body.

Step 4
Rest for a few minutes until you feel like stirring. Open your eyes.

◎ Flower Remedies

Review the following remedies. If any one seems to address any of your present spiritual needs, then use it in conjunction with your movement program:

Holly. To be used when troubled by a negative feeling such as envy, jealousy, suspicion, revenge, or vexations of the heart—states indicating a need for more love.

Honeysuckle. For those dwelling in the past, nostalgia, homesickness, always talking about the good old days, when things were better.

Impatience. For those quick in thought and action, who require all things to be done without delay. They are impatient with people who are slow and often prefer to work alone.

Mustard. For deep gloom which comes on for apparently no known reason, sudden melancholia or heavy sadness. Will lift just as suddenly.

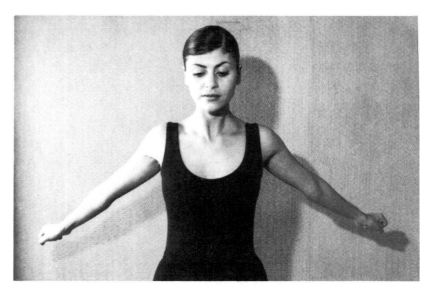

Stretching the Shoulders.

CHAPTER 12

@

WATER BALANCING

Water balancing involves the application of water, either physically or energetically, to correct or prevent emotional and structural imbalances and to maintain and improve overall well-being. The use of water as a balancing and healing tool helps maintain good health by increasing the elimination of metabolic wastes and improving blood and lymphatic circulation. Herbal baths and special showers can increase the activity of internal organs and the largest organ of all, the skin. If you have low energy, water balancing can increase it, if you are overstimulated, water can have a soothing and sedating effect. When combined with Shaman massage and hands-on healing, water balancing is very beneficial when used either before or after a session.

@ How Does Water Heal?

Water is essential for life and is a potent therapeutic agent in many ways, many of which we are not even aware of. Human beings can live for 50 days and longer without food, but in a few days without water, life will end. Water comprises two thirds of the body's tissues. Even a short-term deficiency in water can contribute to many physical problems as diverse as dry skin, poor digestion, malnutrition and dehydration. Water is the carrier that brings nutrients to all the cells of the body and carries waste products. As a healing tool, water can be used hot or cold, as a liquid, a solid (ice), or a gas (steam). Combine water with herbs and other agents, and its therapeutic effects are greatly enhanced. Use it with kneading and water helps to loosen and relax muscles.

@ Water Balancing Can Be Used to:

- Reduce and eliminate muscle pain due to spasms and cramps.
- Reduce fevers or raise body temperature.
- Relieve congestion of blood, lymph, and other body fluids.
- Improve muscle tone.
- Purify the body by eliminating metabolic wastes.
- Stimulate sluggish circulation.
- Reduce swelling.
- Free-up grief and sadness that has blocked emotional health.
- Expand and relax tight muscles.
- Stop bleeding.
- Stimulate elimination through the skin.
- Sedate or stimulate the nervous system.
- Reduce inflammation.

Water has been used as a healing tool throughout history. Sanskrit writings as early as 4000 B.C. report healing baths and other kinds of water therapy, or hydrotherapy. Babylonians, Egyptians, Cretans and Persians used water therapy extensively, long before the Romans left luxurious baths all over Europe. In ancient Greece, the Spartans immersed newborn babies in ice-cold water to toughen them up and to protect them against disease.

The baths were extremely popular in ancient Rome. Galen, a Greek physician of the second century A.D., advocated them in combination with massage and exercise as part of his therapeutic treatments. In the fifteenth century, the Turks popularized a bath where water was boiled and the steam was inhaled as a means to cleanse the system both inside and out. What was known in Turkey as a "hot-air bath" is known in the West as the "Turkish bath." Native American tribes throughout this continent used baths to cure many illness and in Shamanic rites of passage as well as part of village life.

The type of water therapy and hydrotherapy that is used in hospitals and in physical therapy treatments probably has its origins in early nineteenth-century Austria. Vincent Priesnitz, the unschooled son of a farmer, was crippled in an accident, and used water treatments to effect a cure for his condition. News of this treatment and the formalization of various water cure techniques spread throughout Europe and the United States and became especially popular with the royal families of Europe. In 1876 Dr. John Harvey Kellogg, whose brother eventually founded the Kellogg Company, known for its breakfast cereals, opened his famous sanitarium in Battle Creek, Michigan. Kellogg's success was a factor in establishing hydrotherapy as an important scientific system.

My introduction to healing with water came through an unusual process. In the late eighteen hundreds, New York City was teeming with immigrants, many of whom brought the tradition of "going to the baths" with them. There were hundreds of these "Russian" and "Turkish" bathhouses in the city. There were over twenty in Coney Island alone and there were still close to nine or ten in Manhattan by the late nineteen seventies. In the early days some of these bath houses were used to supplement the lack of bathing facilities in the old tenement buildings, but they were also a strong social center for men. Unfortunately, these places were generally closed to women or had one day set aside for them. Most of these places had eating areas where breakfast, lunch, and dinner were served and if it was your day off you could rent a cot and spend the night. You could see men lined up on benches, sitting in their towels, playing cards, smoking cigars, eating kasha, potatoes, fish and sausages and drinking vodka. Among the everyday working people were judges, politicians and a cornucopia of characters, some nice and others not-so-nice.

The overnight sleeping arrangement and the 10 cents a day price tag are gone. Most of these bath houses have closed over the years and the judges and assorted characters have joined fancier health clubs with aerobic classes and exercise machines. But there are still one or two bath houses left, and I go to one of them, the Tenth Street Baths, about once a week. It's the best steam bath in New York. When I'm there I meet a new gathering of healers and those looking for healing through water. If only the old judges and gangsters could see the place now! It looks the same, but the sausages have been replaced by fresh wheat grass juice and whole-grain pita breads stuffed with veggies and ground chick peas. In the baths you can soak tired, aching feet; take a long, hot shower, relax in a warm tub; go in the Russian steam bath, the Turkish steam bath (yes, they're different), take a dry sauna, a whirlpool, go in the hot tub, or jump into the ice cold Finnish pool. It's a real United Nations of water healing. If you don't have a bath house to go to, you can apply the techniques of water balancing by taking herbal baths, alternating hot and cold showers and using vaporizers, and room humidifiers.

◉ Cold Water or Hot?

Temperature plays a key role in water's therapeutic value. Generally speaking, warm water on the body is relaxing, hot water will bring relief to various types of aches and pains, and cold water on the skin reduces fatigue, increases circulation and is generally stimulating to the entire system.

Heat is the most effective technique for healing muscle or tendon strain. This is because heat only affects the skin and superficial fascia. There are healing tools that supply deep penetrating heat and these may be more effective. Penetrating and infrared heat can help increase blood supply along the circulatory root. Deep heat is useful in sepsis (a poisoned state of the system) by bringing more leucocytes (white blood cells) to the area and hastening the healing process. However in areas where infection is not a problem, heat, aside from its soothing quality, is not of great therapeutic value. The value of heat is increased blood flow. In situations where this is not the primary goal, then cold is more effective. In lower back pain, stiff shoulder or knee pain, heat would soothe but not solve the problem, nor would it bring lasting relief.

The effects described for hot and cold water are general and apply to most individuals. There are of course exceptions, since people react differently. Each particular response will depend on climate, the individual's overall health and vitality level, and other personal factors. If you or your partner have any serious medical problems you should first check with your physician before using hot or cold water therapeutically.

◉ Water Temperatures

The following is a guide to water temperatures (Fahrenheit):

Cold: 40 degrees to 60 degrees F.
Cool: 60 degrees to 70 degrees F.
Tepid: 70 degrees to 90 degrees F.
Warm: 90 degrees to 100 degrees F.
Hot: 100 degrees to 110 degrees F.

Once water temperature rises above 110 degrees, the therapeutic value diminishes and can actually have a negative effect on the body (steam is the exception to this rule). When the water temperature is too hot it can cause destruction of tissues, desensitization and dizziness.

Hot water is recommended for relaxing muscle spasms and relieving pain due to muscle stiffness or irritation. It is a good general tool for sedating the system.

Do not use hot water if:

1. You suffer from high or low blood pressure, diabetes, or a heart condition. There is a danger of going into shock.

2. There is inflammation or swelling. Heat increases blood flow and can contribute to the rupturing of inflamed, congested blood vessels.

3. Muscles are flaccid.

4. You are overtired. Heat can lower blood pressure and can cause dizziness.

@ Cold Water

Cold water is stimulating to the circulation and is effective in reducing swelling, inflammation, and the flow of blood to specific organs or parts. It is also valuable for increasing muscle tone.

Do not use cold water

When there are open abrasions. (Neither very hot nor very cold water should be used.) Or when there is a loss of sensation in the skin due to nerve damage of some other condition. In such a situation, hot water can cause serious burns and cold water can cause frostbite, because you will not feel the extremes of temperature. Using extremely hot or cold water excessively can have the same effect—that is, it can cause the nerve damage that leads to desensitization. Do not use very hot or very cold water in cases of diabetes, heart problems, or any conditions involving poor circulation.

@ Hot Baths

If you are new to the art of healing with water, it is important that you keep the temperature within a safe range. If taking a hot bath, the temperature should be between 100 and 110 degrees. Anything above this is dangerous.

Never jump into a hot bath. It is best to condition your body by starting with warm water (about 95 degrees) and slowly increasing the temperature until you are able to tolerate between 108 and 110 degrees.

A hot bath should be limited to about fifteen minutes. If the water cools during this time, add more hot water to maintain the temperature. If you stay in a warm bath longer than 15 minutes or so, your skin may begin to wrinkle. Don't worry: once you are out of the bath, your skin will return to normal.

It is very healing and relaxing to add a few drops of jasmine or lavender oil to the bath or to turn off the light and keep a lit candle next to the tub. This is a great opportunity to practice your diaphragmatic breathing.

Many people use a loofah (a type of natural-fiber sponge), a bath mitt or a natural-bristle bath brush to cleanse the skin of dead cells and bacteria while taking a hot bath. This is very soothing, especially when getting rid of aches and pains associated with muscle strain or diseases such as arthritis, rheumatism, gout, and neuritis.

@ Flower Remedies

After completing the bath, review the following flower remedies and take those that are appropriate for your needs.

Rock Water. For those who are very strict with themselves in their daily living. They are hard masters, struggling toward some ideal or to set an example for others. This would include strict adherence to a living style or to religious, personal or social disciplines.

Rock Rose. For those who experience states of terror, panic and hysteria, also when troubled by nightmares.

Star-of-Bethlehem. For grief, trauma, loss. For the mental and emotional effect during and after a trauma.

@ Relieving Stiffness and Soreness

Step 1
Put on a terry-cloth robe after taking a hot bath, get into bed, and cover yourself completely from head to toe with blankets. This will cause you to sweat profusely and feel weak and sleepy. Stay in bed for several hours.

Step 2
When you arise, immediately dry yourself thoroughly with a dry terry-cloth towel.

Step 3
Gently rub your entire body with a towel that has been lightly dampened with cold water.

Step 4
Dry again slowly and finish by applying a natural oil based body-moisturizing oil or lotion or sweet almond oil mixed with a few drops of your favorite aromatic oil.

@ *Salt Baths*

One or two cups Epsom salts added to a tub of hot water is extremely effective for relieving aches and pains. Epsom salts are an old folk remedy for relieving constipation, but I recommend it for external use only. An Epsom salt bath stimulates the eliminatory activity of the skin and glands and draws out harmful toxins and waste from the body. If you do not have access to Epsom salts, a similar, though less effective approach is to use sea salt or ordinary table salt.

@ *Cold Baths*

Limit cold water baths to about 3 of 4 minutes. They are effective in stimulating lymphatic and blood circulation. This in turn stimulates the entire system. Cold water baths alternated with warm water can reduce inflammation and swelling.

How does this work? On initial contact, cold water tightens the superficial capillaries, driving the blood to the inner body. In this sense it is a counter-irritant. The superficial capillaries then expand gradually with the result that fresh blood returns to the surface. This increased circulation of blood has a stimulating effect on the entire body both structurally and energetically.
Caution: Because cold water lowers body temperature quickly, do not use for long periods of time. If you are a diabetic, speak with your physician before taking cold or hot baths.

@ *Flower Remedies*

After completing the bath review the following flower remedies and take those that are appropriate for your needs.

Vervain. For those who have strong opinions and who usually need to have the last word, always teaching or philosophizing. When taken to an extreme they can be argumentative and overbearing.

Water violet. For those who are gentle, independent, aloof and self-reliant, who do not interfere in the affairs of others, and when ill or in trouble prefer to bear their difficulties alone.

◉ Packs and Compresses

Packs and compresses are a convenient way to combine the healing properties of water with herbs, aromatic oils and other Shaman tools. Packs work in a similar way as baths and showers but offer you more control when you are looking to heal specific body parts. Compresses are best made out of natural fiber and then wrapped within another natural fiber.

◉ More Flower Remedies

Rescue Remedy cream can be used as a topical ointment or as part of the compress for traumatic injuries.

◉ Hot or Cold Compresses?

Moist compresses are very useful for increasing circulation and removing impurities through the skin. Compresses are made of several layers of flannel, often a piece of fabric, a face cloth or a towel cut to the appropriate size and placed on the afflicted area. They can be used either soaked in an herbal solution, used to cover a clay pack or infused with a healing oil. To start, soak the pack in very hot water, then wring it out and apply to the afflicted area, leaving it on for only one minute. Repeat the sequence for ten to twenty minutes, depending on the condition of the patient and the severity of the problem. The treated area should always be completely covered.

1. A compress is several inches wide (the exact size depends on the body part) and long enough to wrap around the part in question with some overlap. The overlap is to hold the cloth to the body either with velcro or with a safety pin. Take the cloth and dip it into very cold water to which you have added a few ice cubes. Fold the moist towel twice to create four layers.

2. Place the moistened towel on the area to be treated.

3. Cover the compress with a dry folded towel, preferably wool flannel when available. Make sure that the dry towel completely covers the wet area, and be sure to avoid drafts. Before you begin the session, you may want to cover the bed with a rubber sheet to make sure that no water gets into the mattress.

4. After about 10 minutes, re-dip the cloth in cold water and repeat the process for 1 hour.

5. After 1 hour, remove the wet compress, dry yourself, and cover yourself fully. Do not expose the wet area too long.

Some healers create a warm moist compress with cold water. As unusual as this might seem, it is an effective healing tool.

1. To apply moist heat to an area, first soak a piece of linen or muslin of the proper size in cold water, wring out the water, and apply the compress.

2. Now wrap this in warm wool flannel. Within about 10 minutes, the compress should be warm.

3. Keep the compress on for several hours or even overnight.

@ Cold Compresses

1. Take a towel or face cloth made of cotton (or some other natural fiber) and dip it into very cold water—water to which you added a few ice cubes. Fold the moist towel twice to create four layers.

2. Place the moistened towel on the area to be treated.

3. Cover the compress with a dry folded towel. Make sure that the dry towel completely covers the wet area, and be sure that no water gets into the mattress.

4. After about 10 minutes, re-dip the cloth in the cold water and repeat the process for 1 hour.

5. After 1 hour, remove the wet compress, dry yourself and cover yourself fully. Do not expose the wet area too long.

Notes:

1. When placing a cold compress on the eyes, use a small handkerchief or a washcloth.

2. Do not use a cloth unless you have boiled it after each use.

◉ *A Waist Compress and Cold-Sheet Wrapping*

The waist compress is a multi-purpose treatment that can reduce fevers, aid in the absorption of nutrients, relieve constipation, improve circulation,and help get rid of headaches. The fabric used should be 8 inches wide and long enough to encircle the waist. Soak the material in cold water, wring it out, wrap it around your waist and cover it with several layers of wool flannel. You can place a thin layer of aromatic healing oil on the skin before you place the wet sheet around the waist. The heat from your body will warm the compress in about 15 minutes and the oil will be absorbed into your system through the skin. A waist compress should be applied before bedtime and left on overnight.

You may need someone to assist you with the cold sheet technique to ensure that you are not exposed to a draft. Proceed as follows:

1. Cover your bed with plastic or a rubber sheet.

2. Take a wool blanket, fold it in two, and place the blanket on the plastic sheet.

3. Take a bed sheet about 9 feet long and fold it twice to make 4 layers. The folded sheet should reach from under your armpits to your knees.

4. Spread the wet bed sheet on top of the blanket. Allow the blanket to extend past the sheet about 1 inch on the top and the bottom.

5. Undress yourself and lie down on the wet sheet. Position yourself so that the upper edge of the sheet reaches your armpits.

6. Fold the wet sheet closely onto your body so that the two sides of the sheet overlap and allow no draft to enter.

7. Fold the blanket around you in the same way, but not too tightly.

8. Pull a pajama top over your arms and tuck it in. In this way, you can keep your arms outside the cold sheet.

9. Pull the regular bed covers up to your armpits, or if you prefer, to your chin. Be sure to tuck in the bed covers all around, even under your shoulder blades.

10. Lie still in the cold-sheet wrapping for 45 minutes. Then re-dip the sheet in cold water and rewrap yourself once again, following the same procedure outlined in Steps 4 through 10 above.

11. After the second wrapping, remove the sheets and blankets, but do not dry yourself. Put on pajamas, cover yourself well, and stay in bed for about 40 minutes.

12. Change into dry pajamas, get in bed again, and cover yourself well.

◉ Hot to Cold Showers

Showers, whether hot or cold, are more invigorating than baths. The flowing action of the water over the body's surface is energizing and stimulating.

One of the simplest and most powerful ways to energize yourself is with the alternating hot and cold shower. This technique quickly and dramatically strengthens the body's vital energy, especially when the cold water is directed onto back of the neck and the genitals. It is an intense experience. The effects are astonishing.

1. Stand under a water shower. Slowly increase the heat of the water till you are under bearable hot water for about 3 minutes.

2. Slowly decrease the water temperature from hot to warm and then colder and colder. You can lessen the intensity by letting the water flow on your feet and ankles first and then up your legs.

3. Allow the water to become as cold as you can stand it.

Remember: Always start with hot water and end with cold. **Caution:** If you have a heart condition, check with your physician before using this technique.

◉ High-Pressure Showers

High-pressure cold-water showers are especially valuable for treating infections of the legs, arms, and fingers. Using a shower-massage unit or a high-pressure shower with the head removed, proceed as follows:

1. Stand in the shower stall or bathtub. Begin with warm or hot water.

2. Stay under the warm or hot-water spray for 2 to 3 minutes.

3. Slowly change the temperature setting from hot to cool or cold water.

4. Run the cold water onto your right foot and leg first, since this is the point farthest from the heart. The spray can then be directed to different parts of the body. This will help you avoid a shock to your nervous system.

5. Spray your body with cold water 10 to 30 seconds; then turn back to hot.

6. Repeat the sequence 3 times. The entire shower should take no more than 10 minutes.

7. When finished, rub yourself vigorously with a thick terry cloth and apply a moisturizing cream or oil.

@ An Intense Approach to the Cold Shower

1. Set the water to coldest setting and spray the area to be treated. If you are using a shower-massage unit or a hose, hold the end of the unit about 3 inches away. Angle the spray so the water pours onto you like a sheet, rather than in single streams or trickles.

2. Without drying yourself, wrap yourself in a dry bath towel and cover yourself with a warm blanket.

Note: High-pressure cold-water and hot-water showers must be used with caution. See discussion under the heading **Cold Water or Hot?**

@ Upper-Body Sponging

For upper-body sponging proceed as follows:

1. In a warm, draft-free room, fill a basin with very cold water.

2. Wrap and tuck a thick bath towel around your waist. Keep another towel handy; you will need it later.

3. Remove your clothing above the waist.

4. Dip a face cloth in the cold water and begin washing the upper part of your body in quick, even strokes, dipping the face cloth frequently.

5. Follow this specific sequence:

Back of the shoulder toward the waist (as far as you can reach, or have someone help you).

Front of the shoulders toward the waist.

Beneath the right arm, moving from the fingertips toward the shoulder.

Then return downward on the outside of the arm.

Repeat the previous step on the left arm.

6. Without drying yourself, wrap the second bath towel around your shoulders and remove the towel from your waist.

7. Now get in bed and pull the cover up to your chin to avoid any draft.

8. After about 30 minutes, put your clothes on, but do not go outdoors for at least another 30 minutes.

@ *Sitz Baths with Alternating Hot and Cold Water*

Great benefit may be obtained by alternating between hot and cold sitz baths for certain conditions such as hemorrhoids, delayed or painful menstruation, low sexual desire, and inflammation around the genitals. The warm water relaxes the muscles around the anal sphincter and relieves spasms. Afterward, the cold water tightens the tissue. Cold sitz baths are excellent for stimulating the energy flow in the pelvis and lower abdomen and tonifying the nerves in this area. They are also helpful for chronic constipation. They are, however, contraindicated when there is inflammation or pus in any part of this area. Hot sitz baths are recommended for reducing nervous tension.

Proceed as follows:

1. Set up two basins—one with hot water, the other with cold water.

2. Sit in the hot-water basin first. Then sit in the cold-water basin.

Note: Repeated immersion in hot water can temporarily impair male fertility.

@ *With Tepid Water:*

Use neutral or tepid water for sitz baths for the following conditions: Prostate trouble (in elderly men), fatigue and exhaustion, asthma, and heart trouble.

Proceed as follows:

1. Stay under a blanket in a warm bed for about 30 minutes.

2. Fill the bathtub with either hot or cold water, depending on the purpose of the treatment.

3. Fill the tub with about four inches of water if you're taking a hot sitz bath and about ten inches if you are taking a cold one. Keep your feet out of the water by resting them against the end of the tub or place a towel under your them to keep them from sliding. A cold sitz bath should last only 2 or 3 minutes and definitely no longer than 5. A hot sitz bath, with the temperature about 108 degrees, should last about 5 minutes, or until the water approaches body temperature.

4. Remove the bottom part of your pajamas. Leave the top part on, but roll it up as far as possible.

5. Sit in the bathtub. Dangle your legs over the side of the tub. Do not submerge your legs or your upper body in the water.

6. Stand up in the tub and shake off the water. Do not dry yourself.

7. Wrap a very large bath towel around your hips and tuck in the ends firmly. Then roll down your pajama top.

8. Lie in bed as quickly as possible. Be sure to cover yourself well to avoid any drafts.

9. Stay in bed for one hour.

⊚ Lukewarm Baths and the Shamanic Vision

1. Lie in a tub of lukewarm water.

2. Add food coloring to the water to turn it sea blue or lavender, and add a candle, soft lights and quiet music.

3. Add a sedating aromatic oil such as pine, rose, or jasmine; or burn burn a similar incense.

4. Then focus on your senses—the sound of the music, the smell of the oil and incense, the feeling of the water on your body.

5. Slowly take 100 long, slow diaphragmatic breaths.

6. Stay focused on each breath and if your mind begins to wander return to the breath.

⊚ Mechanical Underwater Massage

There are various types of underwater massage techniques that can be both relaxing and invigorating.

In underwater massage, the water is directed to different parts of the body by individual jets. This method is most likely to be found in a health club or spa, there are also small units available for home use.

Aerated baths and whirlpool baths are the most common forms of underwater massage. Aerated baths involve the use of compressed air to create bubbles that produce a soothing, light pressure around the body. In the whirlpool bath, small agitators are used to circulate the water around the body.

Whirlpool baths are commonly used in physical therapy and sports medicine to heal tense and strained muscles. They are also effective tools in healing fractures and treating wounds, sprains and paralysis.

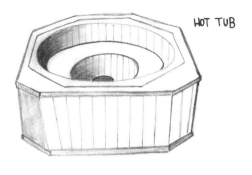

HOT TUB

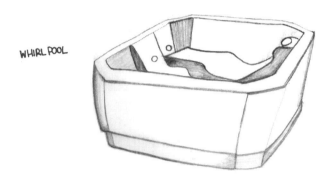

WHIRLPOOL

Underwater Massage.

@ *Steam Baths*

A steam bath followed by a short cold shower bath is purifying and invigorating. When I visit New York City's Russian/Turkish bath house, I use the steam for unclogging my pores, invigorating my skin and helping the body eliminate harmful toxins and metabolic wastes.

Steam is a wonderful tool for relieving sinus congestion and healing respiratory problems. The following is a simple way to accomplish both goals at once.

1. Boil four quarts of water, turn the water off, and place the kettle on a table.

2. And add ten drops of eucalyptus or thyme oil to the water.

3. Sit with your head over it; cover your head and the kettle with a large towel so that the steam will be directed toward your face.

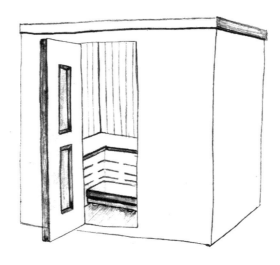

Steam Bath and Sauna.

4. Remain in this position for about 10 minutes. When you first start using this technique, you may need to come out from under the towel every minute or so until you get accustomed to the heat. You may want to stay under the towel for only about 5 minutes.

5. When you have completed your home steam bath, splash your face with cold water and apply a moisturizing cream.

◉ Herbal Foot Baths

I often have my clients soak their feet in an herbal foot bath for four or five minutes before the Shaman massage session. I add a few drops of chamomile, or the herb Greater Celendine. Alternating hot and cold water foot baths is a very popular and effective water balancing technique for tired and aching feet. The water should be placed in a basin or tub so as to cover your ankles and, preferably, reach an inch or two above them. Begin with hot water and soak for three to five minutes. Then put your feet in cold water for half a minute to a minute. Repeat this sequence three times, ending with cold water. When you are finished, dry your feet vigorously.

If my feet are so sore and tired that even a warm water bath won't help, I soak my feet in hot water with Epsom salts added in.

I do this for about twenty minutes. As the water cools down, I add hot water to maintain the temperature. When I'm done I use a loofah brush on my heels and then dry them off with a rough terry cloth towel.

Whichever type of foot bath you use, massage is a powerful way to complete your water balancing session. Apply firm General or Circular Pressure Point Massage to the soles of your feet. When you have completed the massage rub on a small amount of sweet almond oil and then apply cornstarch or arrow root starch. This will leave you feeling refreshed.

If you live in a rural area, you can practice Chi Balancing by walking barefoot in dewy grass or wet sand for 15 minutes to a half hour. These surfaces are excellent conductors of planetary Chi and many Shamans, healers and Qi Gong and Tai Chi Masters can link into it. When you have completed this walk dry and massage your feet thoroughly.

Note: If you experience poor circulation of the feet, use lukewarm water. Although hot water increases the metabolism of the legs under normal conditions, if your circulation is poor, your system may not be strong enough to meet the increased need for blood. Thus hot water may do more harm than good. Be careful in your use of cold water as well. Very cold water can further decrease circulation and can cause further damage, especially in diabetics.

@ Flower Remedies

After completing the bath review the following flower remedies and take those that are appropriate for your needs.

Scleranthus. For those unable to decide between two things, first one seeming right then the other. Often presenting extreme variations in energy or mood swings.

@ Hands-On Healing

Pain is created primarily by an excess of stagnant energy. This energy must be drained from the body or channeled elsewhere. Auricular Therapy (ear acupressure) combined with cold water stimulation is an effective energy disperser.

Step 1
Slow, forceful sustained pressure on the affected points after is a key way of getting this result.

Step 2

Vigorous washing around and behind the ears with very cold water is a powerful stimulator for the entire system. As with the feet, there are many reflexes around the ears that affect the entire body.

CHAPTER 13

THE SHAMAN'S PATH

My Journey

We were walking down a long hill. It was about dinnertime at the end of the summer of 1968. I was very stoned on hash and as we reached the edge of the town of South Fallsburg, I decided that I needed a haircut. I knew there was a barbershop near the pharmacy on the corner and marched in. I got the haircut. I remember nothing about it or the barber other than that there was only one barber in town and he would come to change my life over the years. But I didn't know that yet. It was an anonymous haircut from the man I would come to know as Vincent.

The next time I connected with Vincent was in the heart of the anti-Vietnam war protests. College campuses across the United States were in flux with some being literally taken over by students. I had helped to found an organization called the Radical Students Union and, this being a rural area, we had decided to organize an anti-war march to the front door of the draft board in the next town. I was leading a five mile collection of marchers and slow moving vehicles. I was yelling in a bullhorn as we marched through town and passed the barbershop where I had gotten that haircut years before. Looking at the shop, I saw a man with a darkly tanned face and chiseled features looking directly into my eyes. He nodded at me and I nodded back. No words were exchanged but I made note of his charisma. His gaze was intense. I made contact with this man again through Daniel Norton, a Philosophy instructor on campus.

We all liked Dan. He looked like Jerry Garcia of the Grateful Dead and for a college professor, in 1969, looking like that made him special. Though none of us knew that much about him, we did know that he read a lot of Carlos Castenada, Lobsang Rampa, Rudolph Steiner, Alan Watts and other writers on spirituality and mysticism, and he smoked a lot of pot. I was drawn to him because I had read a book called *The Wisdom Of Insecurity* by Alan Watts when I was fourteen and it had spun my head around. I had been looking for something or someone to grab me in the same way. I thought Dan might be that person. Being in need of a faculty advisor for the Radical Students Union, we approached Dan and he readily agreed to take on the task. It was at our first formal RSU meeting that I met Vincent for the third time.

Dan mentioned that he had gotten a haircut from Vince and as they spoke about this and that, Dan realized that he was speaking with a unique individual with a quick mind and deep insight. He invited Vince to speak with us. It was a revelation. Here was this tightly built, tanned, wiry man of about fifty-five who spoke like a mystic who had done a lot of hallucinogenic drugs. We soon learned that he had never used hallucinogens; he just sounded like he had. Vincent had a long and colorful history in spirituality and politics. He spoke of having been a young radical, describing trips to mystic teachers back in the 1930s. He was a professional boxer: a sparring partner for Tony Zale, the middleweight champ back in the l940s. He described his battle with a brain tumor, a forty-day fast on water that he ended only because his devoutly Catholic mother begged him not to fast longer than Jesus had. He described his interest in physical culture and his friendship with some of the pioneers in the natural healing movement. When he became a barber, he opened a shop in Miami with about twenty chairs and cut the hair and tried to ignore the conversation of various mobsters on their way to or from Havana. He spoke of his serious entry into mystic studies in the early forties and his excitement and interest of this new sixties youth culture. Then he started on us. We had been whining about the military industrial complex and the Vietnam War all evening and he had listened carefully. He talked about the medical industrial complex and how our drug use was undermining our anti-war efforts. He was articulate, understanding and clear about his point of view. When he finished what he had to say, our mouths hung open in awe. He took questions and answered them.

When he was ready to leave he invited us to visit at the barbershop whenever we liked.

I went to Vincent's Barbershop the next day. It was a scene. Though South Fallsburg could not be called a "redneck" town it was not enamored with all the pot-smoking long-haired hippies that the new college had brought into the area. The old high school had been closed down and the local hotel industry, the dominant employer and power broker in the area, had decided to open a hotel technology college in the old high school. With politics being what they were, this hotel school had expanded into a two-year liberal arts college. I had gone there because my high school grades were so bad that no New York City College would have me. So off I went to SCC, Sullivan County Community College also known as Second Chance Community College. I only lasted a semester before I flunked out and went back to New York City. After going to night school for two semesters, I was readmitted. Now I was in this barbershop with about ten other hippies and a few grumpy locals looking to get a crew cut and complaining to Vincent about the environment. Vincent's response to his regular customers was a simple one. "If you don't like my friends, get out!"

As the days went by, I was drawn to the barbershop. Each day brought new surprises. Vincent had an irregular but consistent schedule that he kept in between haircuts. He might be tending the garden he kept in the back of the shop or mixing the compost heap that he used to make fertilizer. It was a unique formula made from a combination of fruit and vegetable peelings and human hair clippings. He kept an apartment upstairs above the shop, not for himself, but to store any one of the drug-crazed hippies whose parents had dropped them on his doorstep. How the system worked, from what I was told by others in our newly forming community, was that someone with a drug problem, mental problem or both would be picked up hitchhiking or on the way to a mental hospital by someone who knew about Vincent. The parents of this hapless child, or maybe the hapless child himself, would decide that any place sounded better than where they were headed, and they would suddenly show up at Vincent's door like the prodigal son returning home. It was Vincent's philosophy that no one was ever truly crazy, though they might be a little looney or on the eccentric side.

Occasionally I would sleep over at Vincent's house. We all knew that Vincent got up early to meditate in the morning and were fascinated by it, though none of us knew much about what he meditated on or why. I once saw a picture of a bearded man in his wallet and asked Vincent who it was. His response was that in time I would know, but this wasn't the time. Over the next year or two I studied all aspects of healing with Vincent. The focus was on nutrition and herbs but every once in a while he might show us an acupressure point or a special way to correct imbalances in the spine. The education was never formal. Vince would recommend different books, or would tell us to visit a certain teacher. Sometimes we would just pile into the car and go off on a drive to visit old friends of Vincent's or an important teacher who was passing through town. Once it was J. Krishnamurti at Carnegie Hall, or Scott and Helen Nearing, the great naturalists and social activists who had built a homestead in Maine. Once when I was on a long fast that Vincent had put me on, we went for a drive to Nyack, New York, to the home of Pundat Acharya, a great synthesizer of Western neurology and Yogic practices. Vincent would educate us on all aspects of natural healing while he slowly made us aware of other realities and other ways of seeing and being in the world.

Once he drove to the airport to pick up an old friend and student who had just returned to America after a long period of study and spiritual practice in Asia. It turned out to be Joseph Goldstein, who has since become a well known and important Buddhist teacher in the Vipasana tradition. Vincent, Joseph and I went into an old trailer and sat for what seemed like an eternity in meditation.

So that's how it was with Vince: Read this book, go on a ten-day fast on water, drink these herbs, meditate, let's take a late night run on the local golf course and pick the medicinal herbs.

As I learned more and more about healing, my hunger for spiritual knowledge was getting stronger. I would ask Vincent about it and he would say something flippant like "Take a Yoga Class" or "Go find a meditation teacher." "How?" I would ask. He would laugh and say just do it.

As winter came, I heard that there was a Yoga class being taught in a church basement in Monticello, a town about eight miles down the road where I had spent the summers of my childhood.

On the evening of the Yoga class it began to snow. Within an hour the snowfall had turned into a blizzard. When I first decided to take the class it was just an interest I had, but now it was more. I had for the first time experienced what is called the pain of longing. Different from an obsession or compulsion, it is a pull from within. I knew that this Yoga class was the door to something larger and I had to get there. I walked about three of the eight miles and finally hitched a ride to the class location. The class was cancelled due to the storm. My inner calling was strong, however, and a few weeks later I did take the class. It was the true beginning of my journey inward. Vincent would direct me each step of the way. He would show me certain meditation techniques, introduce me to different spiritual teachers and share the history of his own journey. He was an "elder" in the true Shamanic sense of the word.

From the time I met Vincent until I took the Yoga class I had been smoking marijuana regularly. I felt it calmed me and gave me some insight but as time went by, this became less and less so. I had begun to develop a deeper and stronger interest in spirituality and mysticism and had begun practicing a simple meditation technique I had read about in some book. Vincent knew I got high and never said much about it, though I always had a sense that chemical or hallucinogenic tools were not part of his agenda as a teacher. I knew Vincent was doing some interesting work with other students and I would sniff around here and there but when Vincent would invite me in I became frightened and backed off. During this time I was was reading various books on spiritual inquiry. The writings of J. Krishnamurti and Alan Watts. During the winter I was working as a waiter in a Catskill mountain "borscht belt" resort hotel and I became interested in one of the waitresses. I was sort of following her around trying to figure out, in my clumsy way, a means to pique her interest. She noticed my interest but didn't really respond. Then one day she handed me a book and said nothing more than "I think you would find this very interesting."

Interesting to say the least. I began reading the book and couldn't put it down. I stayed up all night reading it cover to cover. When I reached the last page the next morning I was completely energized. The book was *Be Here Now* by Baba Ram Das, a.k.a., Dr. Richard Alpert.

This was my first serious introduction to the concept of the world as illusion, altered states and spiritual studies. Alpert had experimented with many hallucinogenic drugs and many students who were working with Vincent had been reading the Carlos Castenada books on his Shaman teacher, Don Juan. I spoke with Vincent about my doing some inner work with mushrooms and plants but he told me firmly that this was not to be my path. Trusting him I took his advice and continued my meditative work. As I continued to meditate I began to experience a pull between the meditation and pot smoking. It wasn't a good or bad thing, just the emotional pulling sensation that comes with resistance. It was as if my meditation was taking me in one direction and the drug was pulling me in another. I knew that I could not go in both directions at the same time. I stopped getting high and continued my meditation.

At about this time Vincent introduced me to the book *Path of the Masters*. The book had been written in the 1940s by Dr. Julian Johnson, a Christian missionary who, while in the process of "saving the heathen Indians," had himself met a Master and had remained to do inner spiritual work. The book was a powerful statement of the inner spiritual path. It was clearly too intense for me at the time, and Vincent supported me in backing away from its message. It became clear to me at that time that I was like a fish hooked on a line. I would be pulled in a little, I would resist and Vincent would let out the line a little. This went on for about two years, when I left Vincent to go to another college. I remained in contact with him on a regular basis and he gave me direction on what the next step might be.

While in college I met a Jain teacher and scholar named Munisha Chitbrahanu. He was a charasmatic soft spoken man who had a great understanding of many of the great classical Indian texts. I and six other students spent a semester in 1972 studying with him and for the first time I felt that I might have met my true spirit Guide. It was the first time that I had a true sense that Vincent was a guide for me but no longer the primary spiritual connection for the work I was to begin. I spoke with Vincent about this and he smiled. With his detached but supportive guidance I saw that "Muni" as we liked to call him was another signpost on my path but not the "Sage" I was seeking.

Even as my studies with "Muni" continued I was beginning to feel that strong inner pull again. I told Vincent that I wanted to begin some form of inner journey. I tried to meditate but found my mind resistant and unfocused.

Surprisingly he suggested I study transcendental meditation as taught by the Maharishi Mahesh Yogi, the Guru made famous at the time through association with the Beatles and later in the 1990s, through the writings of Deepak Chopra.

Vincent explained that it was a simple technique available for a few hundred dollars that would give me some focus and fulfill my desire for some type of yogic or meditative practice. I remember on the day that I went to get my mantra it was raining and I had to hitchhike a long distance. I was late for the ceremony and probably looked like a drowned duck. The sensation of that time seems very similar to the experience of going to that first Yoga class through a snowstorm a few years earlier.

One afternoon, while walking through a school corridor, I noticed a flyer on a bulletin board announcing a lecture in Hunter College's Auditorium with the great mystic, Sage Kirpal Singh. He had a white beard and turban and I immediately recognized him as Vincent's Guru. I went to Manhattan to hear him speak. It was a strange experience. Though he seemed to be speaking in a way that everyone else seemed to understand and was deeply drawn to, I could not understand a simple thing he said. I strained to listen to each syllable that came out of his mouth, but none of it was identifiable. After the speech I was disheartened and called Vincent to tell him what I had experienced. Vincent laughed when I told him the story and explained that though this teacher Kirpal Singh had been initiated by the same teacher, he was in fact not Vincent's Guru. Though they wore the same style of clothing, had a turban, and came from the same part of India, they were actually quite different in style and substance. Vincent was not negative or positive. In fact he said no more about it and I didn't ask. I certainly felt respectful toward Kirpal Singh and yet it seems that it had been shown to me, without my knowing it intellectually, that he was not my teacher.

At this time I was presented with a flurry of teachers. I would see films about them at school or come across books about them. Often I might meet a student of this or that teacher and I would take a deeper interest in each teacher's message. Through all of this, Vincent was my reality check. I would take the bus from SUNY Purchase, where I was now in school, to visit him and we would drive from his house with a few of his other students to meet his friends. Vincent never tried to influence or direct my spiritual seeking but still he would plant a seed here or there by asking me questions or bringing me on a trip with him to meet one of his peers or teachers. That is how I met Dr. Gehman.

Dr. Gehman was a true pioneer in the American natural healing movement. He lived in Duncannon, Pennsylvania, with his sweet wife Agie. I had heard about him for years from Vincent and others. Doc Gehman, as a young man, had been a student of Benedict

Lust, a German Naturopathic doctor who is universally recognized as the man who introduced Naturopathy to America in the late 1890s. Gehman had a huge library of old healing books that he would let me look through and then answer my questions. I felt honored and humbled to be learning from the man who had learned from Benedict Lust. Doc Gehman and Vincent would sit at night around Doc Gehman's fireplace and tell stories about their early years in the healing work. These tales would be mixed in with descriptions about different case histories, how certain client needs were addressed. They would often talk about their friends from the old days: Dr. William Howard Hay, Henry Lindhlar MD, John Harvey Kellogg and other names that I immediately recognized as healer-pioneers from the early decades of this century. Almost thirty years later, I feel as if I was part of some process where the torch is passed from generation to generation.

During this time I was practicing transcendental meditation and following some of the guidelines laid out by Ram Das in the book *Be Here Now*. Then the dreams began.

Over the year that I was away at school in SUNY Purchase, I had been living in Port Chester, New York, in an old private house. I had been sleeping on a wooden floor with little bedding. I call this my ascetic phase. I was fasting for numerous days on water alone and living a somewhat reclusive and celibate life. I had been collecting the pictures of great mystic teachers on my wall. I would look at them now and then to remind me of my spiritual work. Each night I would go to sleep and begin to dream that I was making love. It was a sensual, open and beautiful dream. At the part of the dream where my lover and I were to merge in orgasmic bliss I would look up at this wall covered with the pictures of all these great spiritual teachers. Sri Chinmoy, Sai Baba of Shirdi, Muni, etc. When I looked at the wall, in my dream there was only one picture on the wall; Vincent's Guru Maharaj, Charan Singh Ji. As I looked at the picture intently I would forget the lovemaking and suddenly wake up. There I could see the wall covered with all of those pictures. This dream was repeated a number of times. Each time I would look up just at the point before climax and I would see Charan Singh's beautiful face.

These dreams soon stopped but in my waking hours Charan Singh's face constantly appeared in my mind. This became a struggle for me, as I was practicing my transcendental mediation daily and saw Maharishi as my teacher and yet I felt a stronger and stronger pull toward Vincent's teacher. This pull became so unbearable that I called Vincent asking him what to do. Vincent suggested that I write to Charan Singh directly, which I did. I told him how serious I was about my spiritual work and of the different choices that I had been made aware of. He wrote back a sweet, direct letter. What I remember most about the letter was his suggestion that I find a spiritual teacher without directly offering himself as that person. As to my struggle between various teachers he simply said "you cannot ride in two boats at the same time."

I received my initiation on October 6, 1973, Yom Kippur. This is a day that many Jews call the Day of Atonement, a day when we ask for forgiveness for the transgressions we have committed in the last year. From a Shamanic point of view I have been taught to see this more as a day of at-one-ment with the divine. The initiation process was ritual-free and devoid of anything one might call religion. It truly was the formalization of an inner relationship between the seeker and his inner spiritual guide.

I continued my healing studies with Vincent and my meditation practices through Maharaj Charan Singh Ji. In early 1973 Vincent and I began to disagree about various matters, primarily my view that he was overly rigid and his view that I wasn't disciplined enough. As a resolution to the entire affair we took a drive to visit Dr. Jesse Mercer Gehman, the healer's healer. A health reformer, chiropractor, and Past President of the American Naturopathic Association, Doc Gehman had one of the largest libraries on alternative medicine and healing in the world with books going back to the eighteen hundreds. What I liked most about him was that he, too, thought Vincent was overly rigid. Though Dr. Gehman's focus was less spiritually-oriented than Vincent's, he had a clearer sense of the career possibilities for me in natural healing. Vincent just helped people to heal but never saw it in any professional context. Dr. Gehman was committed to working with patients and thought I would do well in the same format. He also felt that I would have a difficult time making a living at this work if I did not go to some professional school. He recommended Chiropractic or Naturopathic College.

I sent away for catalogues, and as I read through them I became disheartened. My interest was in healing and most of the catalogues consisted of few healing courses and hours and hours of natural science. I wasn't faulting the curriculums. I know that physics, calculus, chemistry and other linear programs are essential to be a knowledgeable physician, and yet the idea of beating my head into intense memorization so that I could become a healer didn't speak to me.

I spoke about this to both Dr. Gehman and Vincent. Doc felt I would struggle without the DC, DO, or MD at the end of my name. Vincent didn't try to influence me one way or the other. I continued to study with Vincent and correspond with Dr. Gehman. I also studied regularly anything that had to do with healing that caught my interest.

In mid 1973 I had read a book called the *Mystic Bible*. This book had been written years before by a doctor named Randolph Stone. Dr. Stone had recently retired and moved to India but I heard through various people that in addition to the strong Shamanic and mystic qualities of this book, Dr. Stone had also written other books describing energy pathways in the body and ways of integrating the emotions, the body's structural elements, and its chemistry with spiritual factors to create a sense of balance and wholeness. His system had come to be known as Polarity Therapy and it was a perfect blending for the student of mysticism, healing and the inner Shamanic path. This was an approach I would learn more about later. At this point I was still somewhat rigid in my approach to healing. I struggled to maintain a regular nutrition and exercise program and though I was seeing some private clients in wellness consulting, I was very strict about combining foods in certain ways or exercising with specific form. Though these ideas were valid scientifically, they were also somewhat ideologically restricting. I spoke with Vincent about my interest in pursuing a progression in natural health care. Vincent suggested I investigate Chiropractic College.

By late 1973, I was driving a taxi in New York City and studying on the red lights. As soon as I saw the light turn yellow, I would slow down and as the brakes brought the car to a stop, I would pick up a book and read a paragraph or two. I would read about a muscle, an herb, a homeopathic remedy or some other aspect of natural healing. Over a three year period between 1973 and 1976 all of those red lights, ten hours a day, five days a week added up to a lot of information on healing and Shamanism.

In the winter of 1975 I heard through the grapevine that an important teacher of energy healing, Alan Jay, was coming to New York. Alan Jay was a brilliant 27-year-old from New Jersey who had moved to California and studied with all the Polarity heavyweights. All except Dr. Stone. Alan taught an impressive weekend seminar on Dr. Stone's Polarity work, concise, clear and practical. He announced that he would be returning in the fall to present a year long polarity training.

When the fall came Alan Jay came with it. Over the next year I studied intensely with him. His knowledge was vast and his ability to integrate energy medicine, herbology and Ayurvedic theory was impressive. It was a very earthy intellectual approach but it was a special experience. There was very little of this type of training available in the East Coast in those days and I felt that it was adding an important dimension to the work I had been doing with Vincent and through my meditation. At the end of the year I was driving my taxi full time and studying meridians, energy pathways and the Chakras.

When I could get away I would go up to South Fallsburg to study further with Vincent. The area was increasingly economically depressed due to the collapse of the resort hotel industry, and had become a sort of spiritual Mecca. Large numbers of Hassidic Jews had gravitated to town and The Siddha Yoga Ashram was quickly buying up old hotels and converting them into meditation Centers. Joseph Goldstein, who had grown up here, had become the leader of the Insight Vipassina Meditation Society and various Yoga Ranches were in operation as well as the sixty-year-old "Vegetarian Hotel." The Vegetarian Hotel would bring up old-time naturo-pathic doctors and healers to give lectures and I often went there with Vincent to have lunch and listen. One of the more popular speakers was Max Warmbrand. In his eighties, Dr. Warmbrand had been an early pioneer in the spread of natural healing after World War I and had been a friend of Dr. Gehman.

One weekend I went to the hotel to hear Dr. Warmbrand speak. What I learned instead was that he had collapsed in New York City while giving his talk and had passed away. The owner of the hotel, a friend of Vincent's, asked him if he would speak on healing. Vincent suggested that I give the talk. I spoke on Polarity. The talk went well and when I completed my presentation an older woman asked if I saw clients. I said yes and so did my first healing session.

When I came back to New York City, I was introduced to Dr. Daniel J. Wiener. Dan was a psychologist with a great personality and a fancy office. He became an important mentor for me. Though my knowledge of healing and wellness had become vast, I was confused about where I was going and was weighted down by a lack of information on how to be effective at life. Dan provided a reality check for me that was to last for almost twenty years. Ultimately he allowed me to use his office which was in the former home of one of the Gabor sisters, and it was there that I began to see clients. Often he would recommend some of his patients to me who where in need of nutrition consulting, herbs or bodywork.

As my practice grew I continued to take various workshops and seminars. In 1975 I spent a year at the Swedish Institute school for massage. I felt a need for training in anatomy and physiology and it seemed to be the most obvious choice. Though I was not a particularly good student, I became friendly with Dr. Sidney Zerinsky. Zerinsky, though never formally my teacher, was someone I found fascinating. An accomplished acupuncturist and physical therapist, he spoke Chinese, both mandarin and Cantonese dialects, and seemed very popular with the fringe, outlaw and lesbian population in the school. He was bright, matter-of-fact about almost everything, with a Brooklyn accent and a New York Jewish quality. He eventually got married, became a Sikh, and moved to New Mexico. I still give him a call every four or five years. His style seemed to have rubbed off on me and I have kept it fondly around my work.

In 1976, just before I finished my massage studies, I heard about Dr. John Christopher from a friend of mine who owned a health food store. Dr. Christopher was a Mormon herbalist based in Utah who had various run-ins with the medical establishment over the years. His reputation had preceded him, especially the news that he had been arrested somewhere on the West Coast for practicing medicine without a license. We were excited when we heard that he was coming east to teach. We were not disappointed. His knowledge of herbs was vast and his teachings were intense. Though most of his information was based on years of clinical experience rather than laboratory research, he opened our eyes to the healing possibilities of plants while his Mormon religious background added a poetic, biblical element to the healing powers of God's plant substances.

Over the next fifteen years, my work expanded naturally as an extension of Vincent's influence and the meditation practice I explored through the teachings and guidance of my Spiritual Sage.

In the spring of 1990, Maharaj Charan Singh died (or, as is often said, left the mortal coil). I would have been devastated but I continually kept in my mind his teaching that the true spiritual journey is within. To worship the physical form of any teacher is to miss the point.

After Charan Singh's passing, I focused more intensely on my own work as a teacher. I explored the integration of Shamanic, emotional, spiritual, mental, structural and chemical factors in living a balanced life and in creating a healing factor for those out of balance. As I became more serious about my work, I demanded a greater commitment from my clients than I ever had before. This shift in my own style and attitude created a shift in my healing work as well. My client base grew smaller while the number of serious students seeking me out grew. I had to struggle with many ego issues, exploring all aspects of the teacher-student relationship. A strong factor in my development in these areas was the teacher who continued Maharaj Charan Singh's work as well as the *Tao Te Ching* by Lao Tsu. The *Tao Te Ching,* after the Bible, is probably the most published book in the world, though it is not as well known in the West as it is in Asia, especially China. This deeply secular, spiritual book helped me maintain my clarity as I expanded my school, The Academy of Natural Healing, in New York City.

When Vincent passed on in 1994, I began to intensely focus my spiritual sensitivities, Shamanic history and technical skill as a massage therapist, bodyworker and healing facilitator as a means of carrying on his knowledge and vision.

Just at that time I met a woman who totally drew my attention away from my healing center. There is no romantic drama or horror story here. However it was the first time I had been pulled so intensely away from my Shamanic work. Over a three year process I began to explore the interaction of my inner and outer relationships. I was about to be be shown the distinctions between love, passion and infatuation. This was going to be an essential rite of passage in my Shaman studies.

Confused and deeply troubled, I found myself in deep pain. It was a pain that Vincent had spoken of—the pain of wanting to love so deeply and yet feeling incapable of distinguishing between love and infatuation. It was the type of pain that people get drunk to forget, or eat double chocolate fudge sundaes to stuff the feelings back down. It was that pain of longing that makes people get serious religion. I don't drink or get high, but if I did, even these could not have numbed this pain. This was messenger pain. A message that you are on the edge of transformation. Of course I didn't know that. I just felt emotional pain. I sat down on my little meditation pad, closed my eyes and began to pray. It was the type of prayer that was a combination "Dear God . . ." and a negotiation. It was an internal dialogue with my inner demons. I explored which of my preconceived notions of romance would I be willing to surrender for true love.

There are certain qualities that I like in women. Certain shapes, forms, fetishes, likes. What would I be willing to accept that was contradictory to these expectations, if by surrendering such expectations I could experience true and pure love?

I sat there creating mental images of the most physically undesirable women I could imagine and asking myself if I could spend my life with this image or that image for true love. I began to separate from the conversation, watching as two aspects of my own personality debated. I was on the sidelines in my own head watching the entire thing take place. The words flew back and forth about inner beauty, personality, style, heart, lust, love and so on. I began to feel deep emotions. Fear, and longing and then fantasies and thoughts of past unrequited passions.

Suddenly, like a light descending from heaven, I agreed that a particular image which I found extremely unattractive was acceptable. I wasn't trying to sell myself a bill of goods. I was honestly exploring my sense of need and the physical picture that owned me concerning desire and women.

At that moment the pain passed and I opened my eyes. There was no resolution intellectually but I knew that my spirit guide had made him/herself known. The wheels had started turning and my process of surrender had begun. What form it might take I had no idea, but I was ready, willing and able.

I drove my car to the health club, about a mile down the road, and took a long steam bath. I felt as if I was floating, actually flying in empty space. I imagined it to be like the sensation a trapeze artist feels just before their partner catches them.

After the steam I drove another mile to a local Yoga ashram to eat lunch. As I got in line to be served, I noticed two large, two foot by three foot sheets hanging on a bulletin board. The sheets had a lot of writing on them and above was a small sign that said "Love or Infatuation." Before I could even walk over to see what was written, I had begun to cry spontaneously.

The "writing on the wall" was three or four pages long. It focused primarily with the distinction between true love for a spiritual teacher vs. Guru worshipping but the message was clear. I wrote down the key points stopping every few sentence to cry or simply thank God for this sweet gift. This is essentially what was written:

Infatuation, conscious or unconscious, is a projection of desirable qualities of your own on someone else. Qualities that you seek to possess, you project and hope to obtain through association or relationship with that person. No one does it to you. The person you are infatuated with is not making you feel that way.

Infatuation is Maya. You make it up. You are looking at your own beauty, greatness, purity, wisdom and placing these qualities on the other person. They may have those qualities, but infatuation doesn't show them to you. You have to free yourself from the need to have infatuation.

Infatuation doesn't respect boundaries. It makes you shameless. Through infatuation, you do not see a person as they are, only as you imagine them to be. Infatuation consumes anything in its path. It doesn't ever respect the person who is the object of the infatuation. It doesn't respect their time, privacy, attention to duty. Infatuation is insatiable. It is all consuming and it will consume you.

Getting over infatuation means two things 1) see the qualities in yourself that you are projecting unto another, 2) see the other person as the fine, independent person they are. Remember, infatuation is not love. Infatuation comes from the Latin word for foolish. It leads to coercion and covert behavior.

Fatuous and infatuation are the same. Infatuation robs you of the chance to experience true love. Free yourself from infatuation.

1) Admit that the good feelings of infatuation is an enemy not a friend.

2) Infatuation is a prison.

3) Infatuation keeps you from doing what has to be done.

4) Infatuation is a trap. It is sticky. It creates the destructive pain of longing but never fulfills. It leaves you empty.

A habit like infatuation takes years to develop. As you age you become more skilled at enmeshing yourself in infatuation. How to free yourself from infatuation? Intake the quality you are projecting on that other person. Until the infatuation passes, take on the behavior of that other person. This will free you. You will get to "be" with the qualities you project on another. You will be with the divine in that person within yourself. You will feel contented and grounded. In that moment, you will see the other person with detachment and respect, and affection which is not hungry."

* * *

At one point I decided that I needed to return to my roots as a healer and that a private, office-based healing practice with a service fee was too limiting in my work. One day, while walking through Central Park in New York City, I noticed a group of about six Asian men and women and one Buddha-like American named Bob. With home-made massage chairs, they performed energy healing on passersby for a dollar a minute. As part of their sessions they might show a client a Tai Chi exercise or a Chi focusing movement. If there was a couple they would show each partner how to heal each other. It was obvious to me on every level that this was the next step. One of my friends and students, Michael Campbell, located a used on-site professional massage chair and graciously drove it to New York from Baltimore for me. I joined these healers every weekend with my on-site massage chair, what I had learned of healing and my healing hands. I soon learned that some of these practitioners were physicians from China, Tai Chi and Qi Gong masters, some twelve- and thirteenth-generation. Over three years we watched, shared and drew generously from each other. I practiced Chi focusing and Qi Gong exercises that I picked up from different masters. In time, when students would approach these practitioners they would point to me and say "go to him, he Qi Gong master." There was always mutual respect and though they did not usually speak English and I didn't speak Chinese we readily shared what we knew so that a large healing circle formed. I could never tell if they were joking or serious, but my hands were definitely becoming tools for service and I felt a level of mastery in my work. I was understanding more and more of the many lessons I had been taught by Vincent and learned internally through my relationship with Maharaj Charan Singh. I was always careful to see myself as a teacher and bodyworker rather than as a spiritual healer. They are different, and the responsibilities associated with them are different as well. In the second year of this "practice," groups of Tibetans would gather just on the other side of the hill and lake that we were working on. They would gather for picnics or celebrations of Tibetan holidays or events related to the Dalai Lama. The combination of this healing work, Tai Chi, Qi Gong, Tibetan celebrations, and boats on a lake near-by created a unique and invigorating environment.

After about three years it became clear to me that my work was being guided to another level. Sometimes twenty or thirty Asian practitioners would line up in Central Park and they were being constantly chased and forced to move along by the Central Park Police who were clearly baffled by the entire phenomenon. Most of the early masters I had worked with in the Park had moved on as well.

At this point I set up my chair every evening on the corner of Columbus Avenue and 72nd Street. I started alone at 7:00 P.M. and would practice my Qi Gong and Hands-on Healing techniques on pedestrians. Sometimes a fire truck or a police squad car would pull up and we would have five or ten uniformed men lined up for their regular massage session. Within another year or two I had the honor of training about thirty-five practitioners in this healing work and they had themselves begun teaching the work in their own schools.

By 1996 it became clear to me that a book that integrated polarity and other energy-based approaches with my healing touch massage and Shamanic exercises would be of great value. I hope you have enjoyed this labor of love and will find it of value in creating health and healing in your life.

◎ Flower Remedies to Support You on Your Journey

Wild Oat. For the dissatisfaction with not having succeeded in one's career or life goal. When there is unfulfilled ambition, career uncertainty or boredom with one's present position or station in life.

Walnut. Assists in stabilizing emotional upsets during transition periods, such as puberty, adolescence and menopause and vision quests. Also helps one to break past links and emotionally adjust to new beginnings such as moving, changing or taking a new job, beginning or ending a relationship and opening to spirit guides.

Willow. For those who have suffered some circumstances or misfortune, which they feel was unfair or unjust. As a result they become resentful and bitter toward life or to those who they feel were at fault. This will open you to being in the world proactively while supporting you in your withdrawal from the reactive thoughts and behavior that will limit you on your journey.

BIBLIOGRAPHY AND SUGGESTED READING

Avery, Alexandra. *Aromatherapy and You: A Guide To Natural Skin Care*. Birkenfeld, Oregon: Blue Heron Hill Press, 1992.

Barlin, Anne Lief, and Tamara Robbin Greenberg, D.T.R., *Move and Be Moved: A Practical Approach to Movement with Meaning*. 1980.

Benjamin, Ben E., Ph.D. *Sports Without Pain*. Summit Books, 1979.

Bristow, Robert. *Aches and Pains*. Random House, Inc., 1976.

Chalmers, David. *The Conscious Mind: In Search of a Fundamental Theory*. Oxford University Press.

Cowan, Tom. *Pocket Guide To Shamanism*. Freedom CA: Crossing Press, 1997.

Csikszentmihalyi, Mihaly. *Flow: The Psychology of Optimal Experience*. Harper Perennial, 1990.

Douglas, Nik and Penny Slinger. *Sexual Secrets: The Alchemy of Ecstasy* New York: Destiny Books, 1979.

Fritz, Sandy. *Mosby's Fundamentals of Therapeutic Massage*. Foreward by Leon Chaitow N.D., D.O. Mosby-Year Book, Inc., 1995.

Graham, F. Lanier. *The Rainbow Book*. The Fine Arts Museums of San Francisco by arrangement with the Institute for Aesthetic Development, 1975.

Harrison, Lewis. *The Complete Fats and Oils Book*. Avery Publishing Group, 1990.

Harrison, Lewis. *Helping Yourself With Natural Healing*. Prentice Hall, 1988.

Johnson, Don. *The Protean Body*. Harper-Colophon Books, 1977.

Johnson, Julian. M.A., B.D., M.D. *The Path Of The Masters*. Radha Soami Satsang Beas, Punjab, India 1993.

Lavabre, Marcel. *Aromatherapy Workbook*. Rochester, VT: Healing Arts Press, 1990.

Lawrence, D. Baloti, and Lewis Harrison. *Massageworks: A Practical Encyclopedia of Massage Techniques*. New York: Perigee Book, 1983.

McKay, Davis Eshelman. *The Relaxation and Stress Reduction Workbook*. New Harbinger Publication, Inc., 1995.

Neihardt, John G. *Black Elk Speaks*. University of Nebraska Press.

Polansky, Greg & Joseph. *Pendulum Power*. Wellinborough, Northamptonshire: Excalibur Books, 1977.

Price, Shirley. *Aromatherapy For Common Ailments*. New York: Fireside/Simon & Schuster, 1991.

Puri, Lekh Raj. *Mysticism The Spiritual Path*. Volume II. Punjab, India: Radha Soami Satsang Beas, 1988.

Puri, Professor Lekh Raj, M.A.P.E.S. *Radha Swami Teachings*. Punjab, India: Radha Soami Satsang Beas, 1972.

The Rainbow Book. Berkeley, London: The Fine Arts Museums of San Francisco in association with Shambala Publications, 1975.

Rolf, Ida, *Rolf and Physical Reality*. Edited by Rosemary Feitis. Healing Arts Press, 1990.

Rosanoff, Nancy. *Intuition Workout: A Practical Guide To Discovering and Developing Your Inner Knowing*. Aslan Publishing, 1991.

Roth, Gabrielle, with John Loudon. *Maps To Ecstasy*. New World Library, 1989.

Sadler, Julie. *Aromatherapy*. London: Ward Lock Ltd., 1991.

Secrets of the Inner Mind: Journey through the mind and body. By the editors of Time-Life Books. Alexandria, Virginia, 1993.

Valnet, Jean, M.D. *The Practice of Aromatherapy*. York: Destiny Books, 1982.

Wood, Betty. *The Healing Power of Color*. Harper Row Publishers, Inc. 1984.

RESOURCES

◉ *Healing Through Music*

Wayne Perry
Musikarma Productions
8391 Beverly Blvd.—Suite 333
Los Angeles, CA 90048
800 276-8634

Mysterious Tremendum Consort and School
P.O. Box 318 Village Station
NY, NY 10014-0318
Artistic Director: Gongmaster Don Conreaux

Biosonic Enterprises
872 Buck Rd.
Stone Ridge, NY
12484

◉ *Understanding Energy in the Healing Arts*

American Polarity Therapy Association
2888 Bluff St., Suite #149
Boulder, CO 80301
303 545-2080

@ Integrating Healing Touch with Movement

The International Somatic Movement and Education Therapy
Association (ISMETA)
148 W. 23rd St.
NY, NY 10011
212 229-7666

@ Bodywork and Massage Professional
Organizations

Associated Bodywork and Massage Professionals
28677 Buffalo Park Rd.
Evergreen, CO 80439
FAX 303 674-0859

American Massage Therapy Association
820 Davis Street, Suite 100
Evanston, Illinois 60201-4444
Phone 847 864-0123
FAX 847 864-1178

@ Shamanic Studies

Foundation For Shamanic Studies
P.O. Box 1939
Mill Valley, CA
94942
415 380-8282

The Academy Of Natural Healing
NY, NY
Phone 212 724-8782

GLOSSARY

Abduction—Movement of a body part away from the midline.

Abrasion—A superficial skin wound as a result of scraping skin against a hard or rough surface.

Acute—Of sudden or abrupt onset.

Adduction—Drawing toward.

Adhesion—Fibrous bans of tissue that help body parts adhere to each other.

Aerobic—Stimulating to the respiratory and circulatory systems.

Agonist Muscle—A muscle in state of contraction.

Altered State of Consciousness—The state of consciousness often associated with Shamans and certain types of healers. These individuals may experience a distorted sense of time and space of time. There is a breakdown of normal boundaries. Intuition takes over in situations where a rational approach was the normal operating model.

Antagonist Muscle—A muscle working in opposition to another muscle.

Anterior—Located toward the front of the body.

Aromatherapy—The use of essential oils extracted from the flower, leaf, stalk or fruit of a plant, shrub or tree to revitalize and enhance both physical, mental, emotional and spiritual health.

Arteriosclerosis—Hardening of the walls of the arteries.

Atrophy—An emaciation or wasting of tissues, organs or body parts.

Aura—See subtle body.

Ayurvedic medicine—The traditional medicine of East India. It integrates many of the key elements in Shamanism and energy-based healing systems.

Autonomic nervous system—The part of the nervous system that regulates bodily functions, such as temperature, respiration and glandular activity.

Biochemical—Having to do with the chemistry of the substances involved in the life processes of any living organism.

Blockage—A limitation of freedom.

Body armor—Patterns in the musculoskeletal system which are reflections of emotional patterns.

Bodywork—Any technique, including but not limited to massage, that involves touch.

Bunion—A swelling of the bursa of the big toe.

Bursa—A small connective tissue-lined sac filled with synovial fluid.

Bursitis—An inflammation of the bursae.

Calcaneus—Bone of the heel.

Callus—Development of thick skin where there is excess friction or pressure.

Cartilage—Hard, connective tissue found at the ends of bones; which absorbs shock and prevents direct wearing of the bones.

Castenada, Carlos—A writer who, beginning in the 1960s, introduced Shamanism to a wider audience.

Cayce, Edgar—An uneducated Christian man who would go into trance states and make unusual recommendations to cure conditions for people that he had not even met. He was so accurate both in his diagnosis and treatment recommendations that to this day people study these case histories.

Chakras—Chakras are energy wheels which serve as the connection between the life force in our physical, emotional and spiritual bodies (Chi) and the unnameable divine energy or Tao that fills the entire universe (Tao). There are seven Chakras in the Shaman massage system.

Chi—Life force. Chi is viewed differently in every culture, moves down different pathways and is generally inaccessible in the traditional scientific view of what energy is. Whether seen as spirit, a reflection of spirit or something else this wireless anatomy is common to all living things. In Chinese medicine, this energy circulates throughout the body along 12 specific pathways known as meridians. In Indian medicine it is called Prana and flows through the breath.

Chronic—Long-standing or recurring.

Collagen—A type of connective tissue.

Congenital—Existing at birth but not hereditary.

Contraindicated—Not advisable, as use may cause problems.

Contusion—A bruising of body tissue without a break in the skin.

Core Shamanism—Michael Harner, founder and director of the Foundation for Shamanic Studies, coined the term "Core Shamanism" to describe the practices of many modern practitioners. These techniques can be integrated into virtually any religious tradition in any culture.

Counterirritant—A substance applied to the skin which produces an analgesic effect.

Cramp—A painful contraction or spasm of a muscle.

Diaphragm—A broad sheet of muscle with attachments at the lower ribs, lumbar vertebrae and sternum, having its action influenced by breathing.

Disk—A pad of cartilage located between each vertebrae.

Dislocation—The movement of a bone from its normal position.

Divination—A Shamanic technique for accessing information about something from "unseen" sources. Some Shamans look for patterns in nature or use divining tools, such as stones, runes, sticks, or cards.

Doctrine of Signatures—A Chinese concept that all things have relationships with each other by means of the similarities they may have in color, shape, aroma, form or function. In Shaman massage this law is applied through a technique called Polarity Similars.

Elder—A Shaman, tribal wise man, mystic sage.

Elements—These are different representations of Chi. The elements: ether, air, fire, water and earth, show up in every domain of our lives and any deficiency or excess in one element will have an effect in one or more of the other elements. The elements are reflected in all aspects of our lives: astrology, meditation, herbs, the emotions, artistic expression, relationships, color, how we communicate, express love, pray, etc.

Emotional Blockages—These are fears or traumas that have stuck with us, often becoming part of our physical being and which limit our effectiveness on every level.

Energetic Healing—Healing by means of the life force that exists in each of us. Also known as Chi, Ki, Prana and Qi, it is the source of all healing. Energetic healing does not require hands-on contact. It works totally on a vibrational or energy level, as opposed to a structural level.

Energy Fields—Vibrational or electromagnetic pathways.

Equilibrium—A state of balance or harmony.

Esoteric—Intended for or understood by a small group of people, often applied in mysticism.

Essential Oils—Hormones, regulators and catalysts which exist in tiny droplets between the cells of a plant. They are extracted by one of several different methods: including chemical solvents, cold expression or steam distillation and are used in aromatherapy.

Ether—That which fills the upper nature of space, or Heaven—a medium, that in the undulatory theory of light, permeates all space, transmitting transverse waves of energy.

Eversion—Turning outward, away from the body midline.

Fascia—Fibrous tissue that encloses, supports and separates muscles.

Flaccid—Lacking firmness or tone.

Flexion—A bending movement which is directly opposed to the normal extension.

Flower Remedies—Vibrationally (Energy Healing) based remedies that have a healing and balancing effect on the emotions and through them physical imbalances. They come in many forms and exist in many different cultures.

Fracture—A broken bone.

Hammer Toe—A condition in which the big toe points upward and the second and third toes point downward.

Hands-On Healing—The balancing of rhythm or life force to create emotional and physical healing. This life force is also known as Qi, Ki, Chi, prana, or vital force.

Hemorrhage—Bleeding.

Hernia—The protrusion of an organ or part of an organ through the tissue which normally surround and contain it.

Homeopathy—An energetically based healing system. Its fundamental philosophy is known as the law of similars, or as it was described in Latin "similia similibus curantur" (likes are cured by likes). This concept of healing states that a disease may be cured by a particular remedy if that remedy produced in a healthy person produces symptoms similar to those of the disease.

Housemaid's Knee—Swelling of the prepatellar bursa, causing pain.

Hyperextension—Overextension, excessive extension of a body part.

Hypertension—Excessive stress and the buildup of tension, causing high blood pressure, headaches, etc.

Inflammation—The reaction of tissues of injury or disease, characterized by redness, pain and swelling.

Intuition—A sense or gut feeling about something. One of the strongest elements of the Shamanic experience is an expansion of intuitive sensibilities. More often than not this "intuitive" information doesn't come in verbal or logical form. Intuition may show up for each of us differently but researchers find that it is generally experienced in three specific ways. These are through: 1. physical sensations (kinesthetic); 2. emotions and feelings; 3. symbols and images (mental).

Inversion—A turning inward, toward the body midline.

Isometric—A way of contracting the muscles while maintaining the length of the muscles.

Kavanah—The Hebrew word for intention–it is often used to describe one of the most important qualities we need to bring to spiritual activity to make it effective.

Ki—See Chi.

Kinesiology—The study of body motion and its relationship to the brain, nerves and muscles.

Lactic Acid—A substance formed in the breakdown of glycogen in the muscles and found in fatigued muscles.

Lao Tsu—A great Chinese mystic. The author of the Tao Te Ching.

Lateral—Outer side, away from the body midline.

Law of Similars—The concept that certain parts and organs of the body are related to other parts by virtue of their similar shape (e.g. the sacrum and the calcaneus, the buttocks and the calf muscles).

Ligament—Band of fibrous tissue connecting and giving stability to bones at the joints.

Malleolus—A protruding bone found at the ankle joint.

Massage—Rubbing of the body for therapeutic purpose.

Medial—Inner side, toward the body midline.

Membrane—A thin, pliable layer of tissue covering or separating body structures and organs.

Meniscus—A crescent-shaped cartilage located in the knee joint.

Metabolism—All physical, chemical and energy changes that take place within the body.

Multiple Sclerosis—A degenerative disease of the central nervous system.

Muscle Fatigue—A state in which a muscle has lost its power to contract.

Neurological—Pertaining to the nervous system.

Non-ordinary reality—The Mental emotional state associated with Shamanic experience.

Orthopedist—A physician treating disorders of the skeletal system.

Osteopath—A physician using therapeutic bone manipulation in addition to other medical procedures.

Osteoporosis—A condition characterized by the loss of calcium from and porosity of the bones, common to the elderly.

Phlebitis—Inflammation of a vein, usually caused by blockage of the vein.

Physiotherapy—The treatment of disease through the use of water, air, heat, massage, exercise and other physical forms of therapy.

Plantar—Having to do with the sole of the foot.

Polarity Similars—A gentle healing technique based on the concept that there is an energetic reflex action between certain body parts. By placing one hand on the point of blockage and the second on its corresponding reflex, the body's healing power is stimulated and the energy is balanced.

Poliomyelitis—An infectious disease, causing paralysis of the muscles.

Posture—The way you walk, stand, and sit serves as a mirror of what is happening to your body and can also be a source for energy imbalances. Remember that what happens to one area of your body influences other areas in ways that might not be obvious at first. Posture is actually the physical manifestation of your emotions, muscles, ligaments, tendons, bones, circulation, and flexibility combined.

Power Objects—These are sacred objects that are often carried by Shamans. These may be herbs, oils, prayer beads, crystals, prayers or any other number of sacred objects.

Power Spot—Certain places on our planet where the universal Chi is richer, where the earth's healing energies are more accessible, more accommodating to the Shamanic seeker. These may include holy cities like Mecca and Jerusalem or sacred mountains and valleys.

Prayer—A call to God, the divine power of the spirit world. Prayers may be directed to spirit guides and angels for help, verbal acknowledgement of one's relationship to the spirits, or a statement of appreciation for grace received.

Psychoactive Substances—Hallucinogenic drugs and plants used by some Shamans for accessing altered states of consciousness. The use of many of these plants is considered illegal in the United States. Certain of these plants are legal if used by Shamans as part of Native American religious ceremonies.

Psychogenic Stress—Stress which is triggered by the autonomic nervous system and is psychologically-oriented.

Pulse—Throbbing or beat caused by expansion and contraction of the arterial walls.

Qi—See Chi.

Quadriceps—The muscle group located in the front of the thigh.

Range of Motion—The fullest normal amount of extension and flexion of a body part at its joint.

Referred Pain—Pain felt in a part of the body other than the part which is actually the source of the pain.

Reflex—An involuntary response to a stimulus, a pressure point which affects another area in the body.

Resistance—The force opposing the natural flow.

Rolling—A condition in which the inner border of the foot falls inward.

Rotation—The turning of a bone at its axis.

Sacred Place—It is a place where you are in the world but not of it. It is a place where you detach your attention from sensory stimulation and turn inward. In this environment your intuition can come to the surface and your angels and spirit guides can make themselves known. A sacred place may be indoors or out, physical or mental. When it cannot be created physically it can be symbolized through language and visual imagery.

Scoliosis—An abnormal lateral curvature of the spine.

Seiza—A traditional Japanese sitting position where one sits on one's heels.

Shaman—Joseph Campbell, the respected anthropologist defines the Shaman as "a person, male or female, who has an overwhelming psychological experience that turns him (or her) totally inward. The whole unconsciousness opens up and the Shaman falls into it." A Shaman may be a healer whose power and knowledge derive from intimate, ongoing relationships with personal helping spirits. Contact with helping spirits occurs primarily, although not solely, in altered states of consciousness in which the Shaman journeys into the spirit realms for instruction and personal empowerment.

Shaman Massage—A series of 14 manipulations and energy-based healing tools based on meditation, acupressure and Shamanic vision.

Shamanic Tools—These serve as the keys that help open the doors to non-ordinary reality. They can include dance, music, flower remedies, mandalas, visualizations and sacred chants.

Shamanic Practitioner—A person who uses Shamanism as a spiritual practice. Any person who practices Shamanism, but usually it refers to someone who has not been trained within a traditional indigenous society. This may include a person in the mainstream culture who has been trained in Shamanic methods and techniques and uses them in ways similar to Shamans, but with more freedom for innovation and eclecticism. These urban Shamans use Shamanic practices to integrate elements of many cultures.

Shamanic Vision—A term referring to what is experienced in a dream-like state of consciousness, such as during a Shamanic journey, while chanting or dancing, or in night dreams. Visionary knowledge and experiences often involve visual imagery but are not restricted to it. Hearing and sensing while in other states of consciousness are equally valid channels of visionary experiences.

Shin Splits—A straining of the muscles of the lower leg, causing pain.

Spasm—An involuntary and sudden muscular contraction.

Sprain—The tearing of supporting ligaments.

Spur—A bony projection.

Strain—The pulling or tearing of muscle fibers.

Structural Bodywork—Any hands-on technique that produces results through the manipulation on bones, muscles or connective tissue.

Subtle Body—Some Shamans and people of great psychic sensitivity can see a reflection of Chi or life force around the body. Known as the subtle body, auric field or "aura" it can reflect physical conditions and emotion states.

Symptomatic—Referring to the indication, sensation or appearance of a disorder or disease.

Synchronicity—A term coined by psychologist Carl Jung to refer to the occurrence of two apparently unrelated events which, together, have profound significance for the person observing them. Synchronicity alerts the observer to the interconnection between interior states of consciousness and exterior conditions in the physical world. Shamans strongly believe in these connections between the inner and outer life and view synchronicities as evidence of spirit activity. (See omen and web of life.)

Synergy—Coordination of muscles or organs by the nervous system so that a specific action can be performed.

Taboo—An object, place, person, or activity that is considered sacred or powerful in some way and consequently around which there are certain prohibitions and requirements. Shamanic world views incorporate various taboos to acknowledge, honor, and respect the spirit and consciousness in various created things.

Temporomandibular—The joint at the junction of the temporal bone and the mandible (jaw), commonly called the TMJ.

Tendon—Strong, Fibrous tissue which connects muscle to bone.

Tendonitis—The inflammation of a tendon.

Therapeutic—Having healing or curative powers.

Third Eye—The intuitive and spiritual center of the individual. In certain mystic schools it is the place where the soul leaves the body during an out of body experience and also at death. It is at the third eye that the mind and soul are "knotted" together.

Thrombosis—The formation or presence of a blood clot.

Trance—A state of consciousness in which a person is not as aware of the ordinary world as when fully awake and alert. Consequently, the attention can be turned to non-ordinary realities that are usually imperceptible in ordinary states of consciousness. There are various levels of trance, from slight daydreaming to a coma-like condition. Shamans use trance-like states when doing visionary work, such as journeying, healing, dancing, and communicating with spirits. (See Shamanic state of consciousness, ecstasy, ordinary reality, and non-ordinary reality.)

Ultrasound—Mechanical vibrations which generate local heat to an area of the body for therapeutic use.

Varicose Veins—Abnormal stretching and swelling of the walls of the veins usually occurring in the legs and caused by excessive standing, obesity or pregnancy.

The Vision Quest—An inner or outer journey. It is a key element in Shamanic practice. It is the process of opening ones inner sense through fasting, solitude, and other practices for connecting to nature spirits so that you can hear the inner voice.

Visualization—The use of visual imagery and imagination to create an emotional, physical or spiritual response.

Web of Life—A phrase that refers to the interconnectedness of all created things. Shamans have a strong belief in the web of life, engendered by their experiences in the spirit world and in their healing practices.

Vital Force (Chi)—Sum total of the body's energy or life force.

Vitality—Life force or energy, healthy and essential.

Wholistic/Holistic—A state in which, in nature, the individual (entity) or other complete organism cannot be reduced to the sum of its parts, but functions as a complete unit.

Yoga—The practice of exercise in various postures, emphasizing the harmony of body and mind.

INDEX

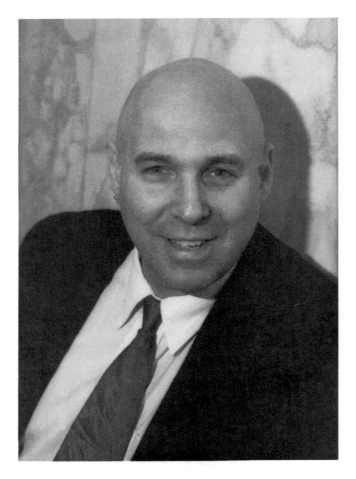

Lewis Harrison is an internationally known Shamanic Practitioner, Naturopath, and Polarity Educator. A Master Massage Practitioner, he is the author of five best-selling books, including *30-Day Body Purification* and *The Complete Fats and Oils Book*. He is a member of the prestigious National Speaker's Association and the American Polarity Therapy Association; he is also former vice-president of the New York Chapter of the American Massage Therapy Association. Lewis's ability to inspire and motivate an audience has made him a highly sought speaker and trainer at major conferences, and he has been a guest on numerous radio and television shows on the subject of healing and personal transformation. He is presently the senior teacher at the Academy of Natural Healing. Lewis may be reached by e-mail at: chihealer@mindspring.com